Body on Fire

A Six-Step Proven Program to Extinguish Inflammation

Vibrant Energy — Rapid Weight Loss — Freedom from Pain — Sound Sleep

Bruce Howe, DC, CCN

Copyright © 2025 Bruce Howe

All rights reserved. No part of this publication may be reproduced, distributed, or transmitted in any form or by any means, including photocopying, recording, or other electronic or mechanical methods, without the prior written permission of the author or publisher, except in the case of brief quotations embodied in critical reviews and certain other noncommercial uses as permitted by copyright law.

Disclaimer: This book is not intended as a substitute for the medical advice of a physician. The reader should regularly consult a physician in matters relating to his/her health, particularly with respect to any symptoms that may require diagnosis or medical attention.

Although the author and publisher made every effort to ensure that the information in this book was correct at the time of publication, the author and publisher do not assume any liability to any party for any loss, damage, or disruption caused by errors or omissions, whether such errors or omissions result from negligence, accident, or any other cause. If you do notice an error or omission, please contact us so we may make any necessary corrections for future editions.

Dedication

This book came from decades of treating thousands of people with health conditions related to inflammation. I am truly blessed and honored to have had this privilege. I thank God for the opportunity.

I want to thank my wife, Julie, who stood by my side through thick and thin during our thirty-five years of marriage. She is my other half, who makes me whole, and she has been a terrific wife and mother to our sons. Julie, I love you dearly.

To my sons, Connor and Slater, who have put up with me as a coach and a parent (and my long work hours), I am so proud of you and your accomplishments. I trust that you will continue to pursue your dreams and always put God first in your lives. Remember that one of the greatest gifts is to be of service to others. I trust you will live life to the fullest and will remember to

> *Dance as though no one is watching you,*
> *Love as though you have never been hurt,*
> *Sing as though no one can hear you,*
> *Live as though Heaven is on earth.*
> *— John Philip Sousa*

Finally, to my family and friends who have been so incredibly supportive and have been a tremendous source of energy and strength, you truly mean the world to me, and I thank you for your love.

Table of Contents

Preface 1

Chapter 1: Inflammation 11

Chapter 2: Identifying the Culprits 28

Chapter 3: How Inflamed Are You? 51

Chapter 4: From the Inside Out 57

Chapter 5: Avoid Pollutants 68

Chapter 6: Choose the Right Foods and Drink ... 77

Chapter 7: Move Your Body More 120

Chapter 8: Stress Less 140

Chapter 9: Better Sleep, Better Health 154

Chapter 10: Smart Supplementation 169

Chapter 11: Extinguish the Flame for Life 185

Notes 189

and dietary supplements had on my patient's recovery, especially when they incorporated this combination with other lifestyle modifications. I was utterly amazed at the faster healing responses and better outcomes that my patients had when they changed their diets and took appropriate supplements.

During the twenty-plus years of my clinical practice career, I have treated thousands of patients. Because I recognized the impact of healthy lifestyle modifications, I was sought after by nutrition-based companies to provide consulting on nutritional product development. I helped formulate more than two-hundred nutritional and supplemental products ranging from probiotics and superfoods to meal replacements, protein powders, sleep formulas, omega-3 supplements, brain and focus formulas, and nutrition bars.

I have often used the analogy that taking care of our body is like taking care of our car. If you've been running your car for years without changing the transmission fluid, the oil, or the brake pads, a point comes when there is a considerable amount of wear and tear on the car. But if you provide regular maintenance by changing the transmission fluid, oil, and brake pads, your car will be in better shape and will run reliably. So, it is with your body.

Today, more than ever, we live in a toxic world. We are breathing polluted air. We are exposed to toxins in cleaning products, in the plastics that package our food and water, in cosmetics and beauty products, and in the buildings that we live in.

On top of that, we live in a society that has been conditioned to eat fast food on the go — food containing more trans fats, more refined carbohydrates, more hydrogenated oils, and higher levels of sugar than ever before. In the United States, the average person consumes around 126 grams (32 teaspoons) of sugar each day, *more* than twice the World Health Organization's recommended daily allowance. Today, many of our foods are laced with pesticides, antibiotics, and hormones. We are ingesting and absorbing those into our bodies.

The bottom line is this: When you combine all the things that you take in daily, year after year, that's a lot of wear and tear on the body. Your body is under constant attack from toxins. You lack the essential nutrients, vitamins, and minerals needed to keep your body's organs and systems operating optimally. Things like poor-quality sleep, belly fat, and chronic stress only make the problem worse.

What's the result? Chronic, systemic inflammation. This occurs when the body is constantly trying to rid itself of toxins, processed food, excess sugar, bad fats and trying to heal itself from continual perceived threats.

So how do you offset it? It takes a whole-body approach, but you can start by opting for a healthier diet and appropriate supplements. The latest research clearly proves the dramatic impact that many vitamins, minerals, and other nutrients have on our bodies: omega-3 fatty acids that are derived from fish oil or plant-based sources, probiotics, vitamins C and D, or coenzyme Q10 are just a few examples.

Scientists are also discovering the benefits of green tea, resveratrol, and herbs like turmeric, Boswellia, and ginger. Epidemiological studies in India, a country where turmeric consumption is widespread, suggest it has one of the lowest prevalence rates of Alzheimer's in the world. Though there are many potential explanations for this observation, a preventive role of curcumin is a possibility.

I never thought I'd become even more invested in learning about inflammation until August of 2016. Despite believing that I was doing everything right, my journey took an unexpected turn.

That month, my life changed. I was diagnosed with cancer. This type of cancer usually affects a small percentage of males in their twenties and not men in their sixties like me: testicular cancer. In addition to the testicular tumor that had grown to the size of a lemon, the cancer had metastasized to an area under my sternum (breastbone) and in the lymph nodes between two major vessels of my heart.

I was shocked, as were my family members, colleagues, and friends. I thought I was going to live to be a healthy one-hundred-year-old because I was doing everything right. I had some understanding of inflammation and the things that it does to the body. After the words *cancer* and *metastasis* from the oncologist really sunk in, I decided to make it my mission to learn everything possible that I could about treating cancer and the significant impact inflammation can have, not only for myself but also to help others going through a similar crisis.

After consulting with several specialists, I decided to have surgery on the testicular tumor, followed by a very intense regimen of chemotherapy for the tumor mass in my upper abdomen. The decision to have chemotherapy was not an easy one. Nineteen years earlier, my sister was diagnosed with melanoma, which resulted in an eye tumor. Her doctors successfully treated it with radiation beads.

Seven years later, the cancer unfortunately metastasized to her liver. Chemotherapy and radiation were the recommended treatments. I still have a vivid memory of a once beautiful woman who'd been left hairless, pale, and emaciated from the ravaging effects of cancer and chemo and radiation therapy. At that point, she had given up hope, and she passed away soon afterward. I had vowed that I would never have chemotherapy or radiation, but I didn't realize that years later, I would face a similar decision.

My oncologist informed me that there was a greater than 90 percent chance that even with chemotherapy, I'd have to undergo surgery to remove the remains of the tumor that chemo could not eradicate. This would require a five-to-six-hour surgery in a very delicate area by the primary vessels of my heart.

During the 120 hours of chemotherapy, I lost twenty-five pounds and all of my body hair. I suffered a number of side effects from the toxic chemo drugs. In addition to chemotherapy, I used weekly vitamin C infusions, immune therapy, acupuncture, massage, and infrared saunas as part of my treatment. I followed a ketogenic diet and walked daily. I also relied on the prayers, love, and support of family and friends. I believe that combining both forms of treatment, traditional medicine, and complementary medicine, was the right approach.

Three months later, at the conclusion of my chemotherapy, the tumor had been eradicated. No follow-up surgery was required. This was truly a miracle for which I thank God, my wife, and my sons, along with so many other family members and friends who surrounded me with love, support, and prayers during this life-threatening time.

I am forever grateful to the medical profession during my cancer treatment. The nurses and doctors who offered their expertise and support were amazing. If it was not for them, I may not have been here to share my journey.

Cancer changes you. I have wondered many times, *Why me, God?* Why did I get cancer instead of someone who was a habitual smoker, an alcoholic, or a junk-food junkie living on fast food? But children and seemingly healthy individuals alike are stricken with the deadly disease. I've come to understand that cancer does not discriminate.

New research reveals why anyone can get cancer. According to a study published in 2017 by scientists at Johns Hopkins, the reason is due to what happens when cells divide and copy the DNA inside them to create two new cells. This process produces *mistakes* or random DNA copying errors that make the cells more likely to develop into cancer. The researchers estimate that about two-thirds of cancer mutations may be the result of these copying mistakes. This may explain mine.

This experience changed me in ways that I did not expect it would. I gained a closer relationship with God, my wife, my sons, and the rest of my family. In addition, I have grown closer to my friends and countless people, many of whom have had or currently have cancer. I count this as a blessing and honor that I have been able to share my experience with them and to support them with helpful information, love, and prayers.

The topic of inflammation and all related things is rather complicated. In fact, many healthcare providers do not understand all of its complexities, which have led to an epidemic of overmedication to combat the symptoms of disease. Yet little advice is being offered by the medical profession to teach patients how to combat the actual diseases themselves.

That's why I created the Extinguish the Flame program and authored this book. The program and the book are the culmination of more than forty years of study, clinical practice, observation, and research. I wanted to create a program based on what we currently know about inflammation, its effects on the body, and the way to combat it, and I wanted to make that program simple to follow.

In the chapters ahead, you'll learn what inflammation is, the reason that it's an epidemic, its impact on health, and its role in many diseases. Most importantly, you'll learn how you can make lifestyle changes to extinguish the inflammatory fire.

You'll also read about real people who have successfully treated several different health conditions by adopting *Extinguish the Flame*'s strategies. These stories are based on my own patients and the patients of other healthcare providers. I've changed patients' names for privacy but have retained the healthcare providers' names.

I'd like to give special thanks to

Drew Collins, ND,

Chantelle DeShazer, PhD, LAc,
Diana Fatayerji, PhD,
Wojciech Konior, MD,
Chad Larson, NMD, DC,
Coreen Reinhart, CCN.

Thanks for sharing your experiences in this book.

I want to thank Bonnie Honeycutt and Kelly James for their support in putting my thoughts on paper and editing the book. They were a joy to work with, and they showed a great deal of patience in working with me.

There is a common thread in all the diseases that come with aging. That common thread is inflammation. The choices you make every day and over time will help determine how inflamed you become and how much of an impact it will have on your health and your life. No matter what your age is, this book is for you. We all need to make a change in this world, and it will take each one of us to do our part. This book is my part. This is my personal contribution toward getting the proper information into the hands of people who need it. I wish you well on your healing journey.

Bruce Howe, DC, CCN

Chapter 1
Inflammation

What It Is and What It Means for Your Body

Take care of your body. It's the only place you have to live.

- Jim Rohn, author and entrepreneur

Benjamin Franklin famously said that in this world, nothing can be said to be certain except death and taxes. If he lived today, he'd likely add inflammation to that list. Not only is inflammation inescapable, but it's also the underlying cause of nearly all diseases today. It's that prevalent and that potent.

Understanding what inflammation is and the reason it's so dangerous is the first step in reversing it. Because while some inflammation is unavoidable and is, in fact, healthy, excessive or prolonged inflammation can have a profound impact on your overall health, life expectancy, happiness, and daily life.

Inflammation Is the Body's Protective Response

Inflammation is simply the body's response to something. It might be an acute or traumatic injury or a chronic condition that has been present for years.

Let's say that you sprain your ankle. Your body responds to the injury by sending leukocytes (white blood cells), which fight foreign substances, to the site of the injury. It also increases blood flow to the area, which can cause redness, heat, swelling, and pain. It's your body's way of eliminating noxious agents and repairing damaged tissue. The swelling around your sprained ankle actually helps prevent you from moving it and further injuring it. The inflammatory response is limited to the site of the injury.

In instances like this, inflammation is beneficial. It's our first response to injury and possible toxins. Inflammation rings the alarm bell, which sends white blood cells to repair and clean up the damage that has been done. Our bodies *need* inflammatory responses to these kinds of injuries. This type of inflammation — a response to an acute or traumatic injury — is a positive thing.

In some cases, acute inflammation can become chronic. If your ankle sprain heals improperly, for example, you may develop scar tissue that results in an ongoing level of inflammation.

Chronic inflammation is the danger. Chronic inflammation occurs when your body's alarm bell is ringing all the time throughout your body. Instead of a brief, localized response, it's an extended, extensive response that affects different organs and systems. Imagine a flickering candle that grows into a bonfire. Left unchecked, it becomes an inferno that consumes anything near it.

Because it's happening inside our bodies, we may not even be aware of the damage that the sustained inflammation is causing…until years later when we start to have symptoms caused by that damage. Left untreated, chronic inflammation leads to a multitude of diseases, including:

- arthritis
- Alzheimer's disease
- cardiovascular disease
- diabetes
- high blood pressure
- inflammatory bowel disorder
- cancer
- autoimmune disorders
- Parkinson's disease

What makes things worse is that many of these illnesses, in turn, fuel a further pro-inflammatory response. This means inflammatory hormones and chemicals in the body continue to cause symptoms that lead to further disease. So, in short:

The more chronic the inflammation → the more damage to the body → the greater the risk of developing disease → the greater the risk of further inflammation.

For example, let's say you've had chronic inflammation for years. This has damaged your blood vessels, and you have developed heart disease. That condition creates even more of an inflammatory response, causing additional damage to your blood vessels and heart. Left unchecked, inflammation can literally be a death sentence.

Yet most of us are unaware that by the time we're in midlife, our bodies may have been experiencing chronic inflammation for years or even decades. The flame of inflammation was lit decades earlier, in your twenties or even in childhood. But it's later in life that symptoms of inflammation may begin to appear.

The Factors Contributing to Inflammation

You now know inflammation is your body's response to something. So, what triggers this response? Some people are more predisposed to develop inflammation than others are. While your genes play a role, it's environmental factors like pollutants, chemicals, and even drugs and lifestyle factors like diet, activity level, sleep, and stress that impact how chronically inflamed we may become. In Chapter 2, we'll look at these factors in more detail.

- *Genetic Factors*

It is possible to maximize your genetic potential by doing things like eating a nutritious diet, reducing exposure to pollution and toxins, getting moderate exercise, reducing stress, and getting quality sleep. In the past, people thought your genes were your genes and there was no changing them. But researchers now know that through something called epigenetics, genes can be altered.

For example, an unhealthy lifestyle may turn on genes that make you more likely to develop cancer. That's the bad news. The good news is that making healthy choices can help turn off genes that would otherwise spur disease. In other words, your lifestyle can impact and even change your genetic destiny. As researchers learn more about how to turn genes on and off, it's possible that they'll learn how to shut off cancer- or obesity-causing genes.

- *Environmental Factors*

Environmental factors include things that our bodies are exposed to, either externally (like pollution or chemicals contained in beauty products) or internally (like medication or secondhand and firsthand smoke). You may not have control over some of these factors. For example, you may live in a city where the air quality is poor. The greater the exposure to these toxins, the more your inner terrain is affected. In Chapter 2, you'll learn more about these common pollutants and poisons and the reason they're so damaging.

- *Lifestyle Factors*

The third group is lifestyle factors. It is arguably the largest contributor to inflammation today. These factors are also the ones you have the most control over. They include the following.

- *Diet*

The *standard American diet* (SAD) typically contains lots of highly processed foods loaded with unhealthy fats, chemicals, and additives and is short on nutrients. Most people consume too few vegetables, fruits, whole grains, healthy fats, and lean proteins. Yet they consume far too much sugar, on average, about two and a half times more than what's recommended. This type of diet is pro-inflammatory.

- *Hydration*

Many people underestimate the importance of staying adequately hydrated. Under-hydration can contribute to inflammation and negatively impact various bodily functions. Water is essential for maintaining proper cellular function, aiding in digestion, and supporting the elimination of toxins. In extreme cases, chronic dehydration can lead to a pro-inflammatory state and exacerbate conditions such as joint pain, digestive issues, kidney damage, and brain damage, and eventually lead to death. (More about this in Chapter 6)

- *Activity level*

We know that physical inactivity is also a major cause of most chronic diseases. It increases your risk of developing heart disease, diabetes, anxiety, and many kinds of cancer. The opposite is true as well. Regular exercise has an anti-inflammatory effect on the body. Yet too much exercise isn't good either. It can produce inflammation, especially when you don't give your body enough time to recover between workouts. For the majority of people, a lack of movement contributes to an inflammatory state.

- *Dental Hygiene*

Poor dental hygiene can contribute to inflammation in several ways. Plaque buildup, a sticky film of bacteria on the teeth, can lead to inflammation of the gums, known as gingivitis. If left untreated, gingivitis can result in periodontitis. This can then lead to more serious gum recession, tooth loss, and systemic inflammation. The bacteria and inflammatory mediators from infected gums can enter the bloodstream, traveling to organs. The end result may increase the risk of cardiovascular disease, diabetes, and other infections. Brushing and flossing your teeth, as well as regular dental checkups, can safeguard against gum disease and inflammation.

- *Sleep*

In this country, we are terrible sleepers. According to the Centers for Disease Control, one-third of all adults fall short of the recommended amount of sleep. A lack of sleep and consistent poor-quality sleep are both associated with inflammation. They also increase your risk of developing conditions such as heart disease, depression, and obesity.

- *Stress*

Stress may be physical or psychological. Physical stress includes taxing your body by over-exercising or suffering an injury that your body must then repair.

More prevalent in today's world, however, is psychological stress. When you perceive something as stressful, your body pumps out stress hormones like cortisol and adrenaline to prepare you to address the threat. This is the fight-or-flight response. That's great if you need to fight off or run from a predator.

Today, you don't have this threat, yet you are likely to be under chronic levels of stress all the time. You're worried about your family, your job, money, your health, or the environment.

We'll talk much more about stress and its impact on your body in Chapter 2. All you need to know for now is that chronic stress is linked to chronic inflammation.

The Hidden Threat: Symptoms of Inflammation

It's important to realize that you may not experience symptoms of inflammation early on, even though your body is being attacked from the inside out. Yet, if you could look inside your body, you'd see chemicals beginning to break down organs, damage joints, and destroy your body's cells.

Once you begin to experience signs of inflammation, however, you're likely on your way to more serious health issues. Those symptoms and conditions vary from person to person, but they include:

- belly fat
- chronic infections
- difficulty concentrating
- digestive disorders, including Celiac disease, Crohn's disease, Irritable Bowel Syndrome (IBS),

- Small Intestinal Bacterial Overgrowth (SIBO), and Ulcerative Colitis
- fatigue
- fibromyalgia
- memory loss
- obesity
- osteoarthritis
- chronic pain (like lower back or joint pain)
- prediabetes
- rheumatoid arthritis
- sinusitis
- cancer
- Parkinson's
- Alzheimer's
- autoimmune disorders

Many of these symptoms and conditions can lead to a misdiagnosis. A lack of understanding about inflammatory responses in the body, combined with the pressure of insurance companies trying to label patients with a disease or illness in order to use a medical billing code, causes doctors to rush and often misdiagnose the root of many problems.

For example, a disease labeled fibromyalgia or chronic fatigue syndrome becomes a catchall for unexplained aches and fatigue. Patients' symptoms may be treated, but the underlying problem is never addressed. Adding to the pressure is Big Pharma, the drug companies, and their distributors, which are continually selling their wonder drugs to consumers and pushing physicians to prescribe (and overprescribe) drugs to treat even minor symptoms without drilling down to the underlying cause. We witnessed this with the Opioid-Oxycontin drug prescriptions for pain that resulted in overdoses, thousands of deaths, and billions of dollars in lawsuits.

Treating Inflammation from the Inside Out

So what's the answer? It's not prescribing more drugs. It starts with understanding the process of chronic inflammation and doing what you can to stop it.

In my twenty-one years of clinical practice, I saw patients who had been diagnosed with headaches, heart disease, and diabetes. I've also treated people with severe arthritis and autoimmune diseases. These patients were all dealing with life-changing conditions. Yet most of them were unaware that inflammation was the likely root cause of their medical issues, nor did they understand how they could potentially reverse it.

Just as concerning is the fact that I've also seen more and more depression in individuals, particularly in young people who are struggling to cope with the stressors of day-to-day life. This kind of unrelenting stress can lead to depression, anxiety, and even suicide.

Depression in Teens Is a Growing Problem

Today's teens are more likely to be depressed than ever before. According to the National Institute of Mental Health (NIMH), one in five teens will experience major depression before reaching adulthood, yet less than one-third of them are treated for depression. This is one reason why, every one hundred minutes, a teen takes his or her own life. In fact, suicide is the third-leading cause of death for people between the ages of fifteen and twenty-four.

New research has found a link between cell phone use and other digital screen media technology, which affects brain chemicals called neurotransmitters, and depression among teens. The more hours teens spend on their phones and other screen media, the more likely they are to be depressed and have suicidal thoughts.

> If you have a teenaged child or grandchild, don't assume that his or her mood changes, loss of interest in activities, or social isolation are normal for adolescents, they may be cries for help. Let him or her know that you care and take the necessary steps to get your teen help and treatment, which may include counseling, medical care, and nutritional support.

During my years of clinical practice, I didn't merely take a comprehensive history and conduct a physical examination to diagnose the root cause of an individual's symptoms. If I thought it was warranted, based on the patient's history and examination, I would do a more extensive evaluation, including laboratory tests that were a combination of blood, urine, stool, and saliva testing for certain biomarkers. For example, C-reactive protein is one of the most common measures of inflammation in the body. A simple blood test provides an important indication of how inflamed someone is. In Chapter 4, you'll learn more about the tests you can take to determine how inflamed your body is.

In many cases, people who had chronic pain or compromised immune function had some type of digestive disorder as well. For example, Eva was an eighty-one-year-old woman who had chronic joint pain. She had also been diagnosed with diverticulitis, a severe digestive condition where portions of her intestinal lining had become inflamed over time. Eva had been scheduled to have surgery to remove more than one-third of her colon. In addition to the dangers of surgery, she may have suffered excessive blood loss, difficulty in healing after surgery, and a possible bowel obstruction afterward. She wanted to try another approach.

We determined that her inflammatory markers were elevated. She also tested positive for gluten intolerance and other food sensitivities. After evaluating her diet, she agreed to try an allergy-free diet, one that eliminated wheat, gluten, soy, dairy, and nightshade vegetables, which were foods that

I believed were contributing to her issues. I also suggested that she take gut-healing supplements like glutamine, digestive enzymes, prebiotics, probiotics, and other natural botanicals.

Within three months, all of her symptoms had disappeared, and her surgery was canceled. Although Eva was fighting decades of inflammation, simply changing her diet and having her take the right kind of supplements turned her life around.

I've seen numerous patients with what they thought were chronic conditions they had to live with — things like arthritis, celiac disease, Crohn's disease, and autoimmune conditions like fibromyalgia — improve their symptoms and overall health when they made lifestyle changes. The same is true with many of my forward-thinking colleagues in health care, some of whom have shared their patients' experiences in this book.

Traditional medicine, at times, can be miraculous and offer life-changing solutions; however, often, it is quick to offer medication to treat symptoms, yet it's better to treat the underlying cause instead, which is often inflammation. Over the years, I have seen patients with a variety of headaches. Upon examination and evaluation, if appropriate, I have provided chiropractic care to help remove structural imbalance and nerve interference. In many cases, I have also recommended a diet that eliminates inflammatory foods like gluten, dairy, soy, sugar, artificial sweeteners, alcohol, excessive caffeine intake, and other potential allergens and the reduction of stress. In nearly every case, the headaches and migraines were alleviated within a couple of months. It should be noted that there is a National Institutes of Health (NIH) classification of headaches that supports a rational alternative for other forms of treatment than what I have addressed.

> ### *Treating Celiac Disease with Dietary Changes*
>
> Mark had previously been diagnosed with celiac disease, an inflammatory disease of the colon that leaves you unable to digest gluten, a protein found in many grains. Mark, 41, avoided gluten "90 percent of the time" but still complained of low energy, heartburn, diarrhea, and itchy skin. Testing revealed that his liver enzymes were elevated, as was his C-reactive protein (a marker of inflammation.) He was also low in vitamin D and had high cholesterol.
>
> Four weeks after switching to a low-allergen, anti-inflammatory diet, Mark's diarrhea was gone. His heartburn symptoms had eased. He had more energy, and his skin had improved. A bonus? He had lost a significant amount of weight. Testing confirmed that his markers of inflammation and toxicity were significantly improved.
>
> Eliminating possible trigger foods was all he needed to do to quell inflammation, and get on the path to better health.
>
> - Diana Fatayerji, PhD

Is a Gluten-Free Diet Right for You?

Twenty-five years ago, long before going gluten-free became a trend, I was recommending gluten-free diets to my patients who had unexplained gut symptoms like bloating, abdominal pain, diarrhea, and constipation. I personally had some unexplained gastrointestinal (GI) issues and what is called atopic dermatitis (unexplained skin rashes). The dermatologist's only recommendation was to use cortisone cream.

But when I experimented with an elimination diet, eating more organic foods not laced with chemicals, like glyphosate (AKA Roundup), antibiotics, and cutting out gluten, I discovered that my symptoms had disappeared, never to recur. It's been my experience that many people with gut problems, skin issues, joint pain, and a variety of other conditions often have gluten intolerance or sensitivity. When they stop consuming gluten chemically laden processed foods and cut back on sugar, their symptoms clear up.

Back then, I was told by so-called medical experts that gluten-free was simply a fad. Today, however, more people are eliminating gluten from their diets and finding that their health improves. The medical community as a whole is finally taking notice.

The fact is that food allergies and sensitivities contribute to inflammation. Yet millions of people are unaware of their sensitivities. They are making their inflammation worse because they are consuming foods that their bodies can't properly digest. If you have these kinds of symptoms, eliminating gluten or other common allergens may be the answer (things like dairy products, soy, eggs, nuts, and, although not an allergen, one of the biggest culprits, sugar).

Is Inflammation the Culprit Behind Chronic Headaches?

Ashlee was only 15 when she sought help for congestion and the chronic sinus headaches she'd been dealing with since she was a baby. She always felt tired and had extreme difficulty focusing, so school was challenging.

Ashlee started drinking more water and followed an anti-inflammatory diet that was free of gluten, soy, and dairy products and low in sugar. In addition to receiving acupuncture, she took supplements, including green superfoods, omega fish oil, plant protein, and a supplement with botanicals such as turmeric, ginger, and Boswellia.

Within two weeks, she had more energy and could complete her homework easily. Several months later, she says she can't remember the last time she had a headache

> and no longer wakes up in the morning worried about whether she'll have one. She not only feels better, she feels more confident about her life overall. That's how a teenager should feel.
>
> - Chantelle DeShazer, PhD, LAc

The Inflammation Answer: The Extinguish the Flame Program

Chronic inflammation is an epidemic. People are living with inflammation, often without knowing it. They don't know how to reverse it — to squelch the bonfire until it is a more manageable, smaller, and healthier flame. Over the decades as a health care practitioner and certified clinical nutritionist working with thousands of patients and researching what works (and what doesn't), I've developed the *Extinguish the Flame Program*.

The *Extinguish the Flame Program* includes six simple steps to extinguish the flame.

- *Changing Your Environment*

Reduce your exposure to toxins and pollutants when you can.

- *Eating*

Focus on eating whole, nutritious foods in their natural states while limiting or eliminating processed foods, reducing sugar, and other inflammation triggers.

- *Moving*

Add the right amount of activity to your life, or in some cases, adapt your exercise program to produce minimal inflammation.

- *Stress Busting*

Learn how to manage stress better, which includes adding more playtime to your life, laughing and loving more, and expressing gratitude more often. I also recommend seeing a counselor when appropriate.

- *Sleeping*

Learn how to get optimal sleep, in quality and quantity, to let your body function at its best.

- *Supplementing*

Learn which supplements can help reduce inflammation and the way they work in conjunction with a healthy diet to maximize your body's performance.

What's the bad news? As you've seen, some chronic inflammation is inescapable. The good news is that inflammation can be controlled and, depending on your health, even reversed. I have personally witnessed this in the countless people that I've worked with over the years. People who had to take drugs to treat high blood pressure or diabetes were able to eliminate them as their overall health improved (Don't stop taking any medication that you are currently on without talking to your healthcare provider first).

However, it is important to note that there are two types of diabetes. People with type 1 diabetes produce no insulin, and their condition cannot be altered by supplements. In contrast, those with type 2 diabetes have a different situation; their condition can be improved with supplements and other interventions.

As a nation, we're indoctrinated and programmed by the media to believe that taking a pill will fix the situation — there's a drug or many drugs for every disease. Yet, often, medication doesn't address the underlying problem, and it may cause side effects and other problems.

For example, my eighty-five-year-old sister, Mary, developed plantar fasciitis several years ago. She also has heel spurs on the bottoms of her feet, which can cause additional inflammation of the plantar fascia (the connective tissue that runs along the soles of your feet). You can treat this condition with exercise, stretching the calf muscles, massage, certain types of laser treatment, and ultrasound.

But that only addresses the symptoms. What's the underlying culprit here? An inflammatory process is at work, which has been most likely caused by an improper gait, which leads to mechanical stress on the bones and soft tissues of the feet.

Incorporating a combination of massage, stretching, and an anti-inflammatory diet (consuming more fruits and vegetables loaded with alkaline minerals like magnesium and potassium), taking natural anti-inflammatory supplements like fish oil, turmeric, Boswellia, and ginger, resveratrol, quercetin, and applying some patience will lead to a successful recovery. In some cases, it may be necessary to get foot orthotics to improve one's gait.

A lifetime of an inflammatory lifestyle can take quite a toll. My mother lived to the ripe old age of ninety-three. Although her mind was sharp as a tack, she suffered from severe osteoporosis (bone loss) and had multiple spinal compression fractures, which resulted in a loss of six inches in height.

She loved to bake, and white flour and sugar were at the top of her ingredients list. She also loved her meats, cold cuts, cheese, white bread, and crackers. She did not like brightly colored fruits, vegetables, and dark leafy greens, which are all anti-inflammatory foods. She also drank one to two pots of coffee daily. The combination of a highly acidic diet along with a hormonal imbalance (most likely from being pregnant eight times) was the underlying cause of her bone loss.

Whether you're already starting to have symptoms of inflammation like those discussed earlier or you simply want to ensure you live the healthiest, happiest, longest life you can, the *Extinguish the Flame Program* is the answer.

Preparing to Extinguish the Flame

What is my promise to you? You can give your body a chance to reset a chronic inflammatory response with this program. I know that it's normal to resist making any kind of lifestyle modification, whether it's changing your diet or exercising differently. Many people may not be willing to change until their symptoms are causing pain or they are experiencing significant health consequences. The more severe the problem, the more motivated the person may be to change. That's because we live in a world where most people want immediate gratification and quick-fix solutions.

It's easy to think that little things like a salad dressing containing trans fats aren't a big deal, but little things add up. The effects are cumulative. When you're consuming a *little bit* of salad dressing or other trans fats (found in fried foods, baked goods, and restaurant fare), frequently or even occasionally, over the years, it all makes a difference.

The opposite is true as well. Establishing new micro-habits and making small adjustments like swapping out your usual salad dressing for olive oil and apple cider vinegar or fresh lemon juice will help in the long run. Just as bad foods or choices have a cumulative effect, good foods and positive changes do too. Each one matters.

Let's say you eat out a lot, regularly order fast food like burgers and fries, and enjoy eating this way. Sure, it would be better if you swapped out all junk food, but making some small changes, like ordering a side salad instead of fries or ordering a grilled chicken sandwich, are steps in the right direction. Some people really struggle with making drastic lifestyle changes, so if baby steps work better for you, that's fine.

What's my point? Even if you can't or don't follow every recommendation in the *Extinguish the Flame Program*, every small change you make will help reduce inflammation in your body and improve your health. This book is meant to be your guide and not your taskmaster. So pay attention. Experiment with what works for you and what doesn't.

Finally, there's a tendency to think of being healthy as simply avoiding disease, but I encourage you to think more broadly than that. When you know the reason why inflammation occurs and the way to manage it, you can not only reduce your risk of developing conditions like heart disease, diabetes, asthma, arthritis, and high blood pressure but also improve your overall health. You can also change and improve the way you feel each day in terms of steadier energy levels, higher productivity levels, easier management of stress, better sleep, and an improved positive mood.

In short, reducing inflammation can improve your here and now and your future, as well. So let's get started!

Chapter 2
Identifying the Culprits

The Causes of Chronic Inflammation

Living in this modern toxic world, we are all slowly being poisoned to death.

- Carrie Latet, Diet Diva chef and author

As you saw in Chapter 1, there are three primary contributors to chronic inflammation: genetic factors, environmental factors, and lifestyle factors. Understanding what these factors are and how prevalent they are in our modern world will convince you of the necessity of doing what you can to combat inflammation.

Genetic Factors Affecting Inflammation

In short, genetic factors refer to the genes you were born with. Some people are simply more susceptible to chronic inflammation than others are. It's important to note that the way you choose to live in terms of your diet, the amount of sleep you get, and the way you manage stress can have a significant impact on whether certain genes get turned on or activated. We won't spend much time discussing genetic factors because when you make positive lifestyle changes like the ones in the *Extinguish the Flame Program*, you'll help turn on healthy genes and shut off unhealthy ones.

There are some factors that you can't control. New research has found that about two-thirds of cancers may be caused by genetic copying mistakes that occur when the body's cells divide (more about that in Chapter 11).

Environmental Factors Contributing to Inflammation

New research from the UC Berkeley School of Public Health shows that childhood exposure to the world's most widely used weed killer, glyphosate, is linked to liver inflammation and metabolic disorders in early adulthood, which could lead to liver cancer, diabetes, and cardiovascular disease later in life.

Some environmental factors are pesticides, herbicides, household cleaners, perfumes, food additives, flame-retardant materials, and plastics. Our shampoos and cosmetics are laden with fungicides and bactericides called parabens or, more precisely, parahydroxy-benzoates. Our deodorant contains aluminum as well as parabens. Glyphosate, also known as Roundup, a popular herbicide used worldwide, has been shown to infiltrate the brain, resulting in inflammation.

According to the Civil Eats online publication dated March 22, 2024

> Paraquat, an herbicide also used to control weeds that glyphosate does not control, has been and still is one of the most popular herbicides in the U.S. Paraquat is applied in the greatest quantities to fields of soybeans, cotton, and grapes, according to the U.S. Geological Survey. It's also the deadliest pesticide used in U.S. agriculture, capable of killing a human with just a sip, as the U.S. Environmental Protection Agency (EPA) warns. As far back as 1983, journalist Andrew Revkin warned that "the potent weedkiller is killing people," as he starkly detailed its link to suicides and accidental deaths. A considerable body of evidence links the toxicant to Parkinson's disease, a progressive neurological condition with no cure.

Observing these dangers to life and health, more than 50 countries have now banned paraquat, including the E.U., the

U.K., China, and Brazil. Despite longtime calls for the EPA to ban paraquat, it remains legal on U.S. farms if those who apply it receive certified training, and it is often applied by farmworkers who have no say over its use. Yet, the next couple of years could prove to be critical for the future of paraquat, which has fallen under sharper scrutiny as it faces a growing number of legal challenges.

Our homes, schools, and offices are built using materials that contain formaldehyde, which is a main agent in the embalming fluid that is used to preserve dead bodies. In many cases, we're wiping it all over our faces as it's also used as a wet-strength resin in facial tissue, napkins, and paper towels. In 2011, the US National Toxicology Program declared formaldehyde to be a human carcinogen.

Gas ranges, if not well-vented, can produce toxic amounts of nitrogen dioxide, which leads to respiratory problems. Then there's air pollution, secondhand smoke, smog, exhaust fumes, and on and on and on.

Our bodies are suffocating. These chemicals and toxins contribute greatly and silently to chronic inflammation and toxicity. We can see its effects: allergies, asthma, bronchitis, contact dermatitis, psoriasis, liver disease, kidney failure, and cancer.

Everything you eat or drink has to be processed by your organs and ends up in your bloodstream. Every breath you take has to be processed by your lungs and ends up in your bloodstream. Everything you put on your body — deodorant, shampoo, soap, body wash, bubble bath, facial moisturizer, toner, cosmetics, lotion, perfume, sunscreen, detergent used in laundry — is absorbed through your skin and ends up in your bloodstream.

Don't become overwhelmed and simply give up because there is much hope. As you'll see in Chapter 4, our bodies are fantastic, miraculous filtration machines. Your lungs, liver, kidneys, and other sophisticated systems work together to capture the toxins and release them through your breath, intestinal system, and urinary tract.

Yet problems can and do occur when your system becomes so overloaded it can't work efficiently. Our goal with the *Extinguish the Flame Program* is to help you learn how to unburden your body's own system. In Chapter 5, you'll learn how to lessen the impact of a toxic environment.

Lifestyle Factors Contributing to Inflammation

There are several lifestyle factors impacting your body's likelihood of chronic inflammation, and they all play a powerful role. They include:

- central adiposity, what we commonly call belly fat (This can be both a lifestyle factor and the result of a pro-inflammatory diet)
- a diet that includes a lot of overly processed foods, too much sugar, and few of the whole foods that provide the nutrients our bodies need
- excess alcohol consumption
- overuse of antibiotics
- certain over-the-counter (OTC) and prescription medications
- a lack of physical activity
- an inability to manage stress
- a lack of quality sleep

You can see that these factors influence each other. For example, consuming too much sugar makes you more likely to be overweight and to have belly fat, which makes inflammation worse. If you're stressed by your day and aren't sleeping, you again have two factors contributing to inflammation. Let's look at each of these in turn.

- *Central Adiposity*

Central adiposity, what we commonly call belly fat, is a red flag for inflammation. According to researchers, there's a direct correlation between the amount of belly fat a person has and his or her susceptibility to encountering cardiovascular disease (heart attack and stroke), insulin resistance and type 2 diabetes, colorectal cancer, sleep apnea, high blood pressure, degenerative diseases, and premature death, just to name a few.

When it comes to body fat, not all fat is equal. There are actually two types of fat in your abdominal area. One is the kind of *subcutaneous fat* that lies just under your skin and on top of your muscles, covering your abs and keeping that six-pack from being visible. This is *vanity fat*. You may not like how it looks, but it's not particularly dangerous when it comes to producing an inflammatory response.

The second type of fat, *visceral fat*, is the more dangerous of the two. Visceral fat lies much deeper, below the abdominal muscles, and surrounds the internal organs. Visceral belly fat releases inflammatory molecules into your body's bloodstream on a continual basis. The more belly fat you have, the more toxic flooding is happening (twenty-four hours a day) and creating a vicious cycle that keeps you fat and inflamed.

This fat doesn't just sit there padding your internal organs. It acts as another organ in your body, secreting chemicals and hormones that, in turn, can raise your cortisol levels and impact your hormone and immune functions (We'll talk more about cortisol and the stress response later in this chapter).

Does this mean you need to do hundreds of sit-ups daily in order to get rid of your belly fat? No. In fact, that kind of spot reduction doesn't work. The only way to reduce belly fat is to follow a healthy, inflammation-reducing diet and move your body more so that you burn more calories than you consume.

Having some body fat is good. Body fat helps maintain healthy skin and hair, ensures the smooth functioning of cells, helps maintain body temperature, stores energy, and helps absorb essential nutrients. However, too much fat sets off a domino effect in the body and triggers bad hormones to flood the body and good hormones to stop their production. What is the end result? Obesity, inflammation, and disease.

If you are overweight, every little bit of extra fat you eliminate makes a difference. If you lose one pound of fat, that's one less pound that will contribute to raising your insulin and cortisol levels. That's one less pound to cause strain on your internal organs. That's one less pound to cause stress on your joints. Research shows that losing just 5 or 10 percent of your body weight can significantly improve your health and reduce your risk of developing diabetes.

The key is to avoid becoming overwhelmed by the amount of fat that you need to lose. Focus on making slow, steady progress each week (By the way, having trouble with losing weight is yet another sign of inflammation). Ignore the advertisements that tout astounding stories of losing five to ten pounds within a week or more. That is not only unreasonable but unhealthy. The recommended safe rate of weight loss is one to two pounds per week. Any more than that can be dangerous to your health. The *Extinguish the Flame Program* will help you achieve this kind of healthy, sustainable weight loss.

When You Can't Lose Weight: Bella's Story

Like many women, Bella was overweight, yet she could not shed the pounds. The 28-year-old was extremely fatigued. Her lab tests revealed she had hyperlipidemia (high cholesterol and triglycerides), low vitamin D, gluten sensitivity, and a significantly elevated C-reactive protein, a biomarker that measures the amount of inflammation.

Bella was prescribed an anti-inflammatory, gluten-free diet that included quality proteins, leafy greens, non-starchy vegetables, and some fruits and berries. She cut all grains, sweets, and junk food from her diet and took high-potency fish oil, curcumin, vitamin D, a ketone salt

> Bella was prescribed an anti-inflammatory, gluten-free diet that included quality proteins, leafy greens, non-starchy vegetables, and some fruits and berries. She cut all grains, sweets, and junk food from her diet and took high-potency fish oil, curcumin, vitamin D, a ketone salt product, and a high-quality multi-vitamin. Within a few months, her energy had increased significantly, she had lost weight, and her clothes were fitting better. Testing revealed her vitamin D, cholesterol, triglycerides, and CRP were all now in optimal range. Best of all? She says, "I feel like myself again."
>
> - Chad Larson, NMD

While there are various methods to measure body fat accurately, some simple and accessible ways to estimate body fat at home include:

- Body Fat Calipers:
    - Body fat calipers are affordable and easy to use. They measure skinfold thickness at different points on the body. You can find guidelines online to ensure accurate measurements. Keep in mind that technique and consistency are crucial for reliable results.

- Bioelectrical Impedance Analysis (BIA) Scales:
    - BIA scales send a low electrical current through the body to estimate body fat percentage. While these scales are convenient, factors like hydration levels can affect accuracy. Follow the instructions carefully and measure at the same time each day for consistency.

- Online Calculators:
    - Various online calculators use measurements like waist circumference, height, weight, and, sometimes, hip circumference to estimate

body fat percentage. These calculations provide a rough estimate and may not be as accurate as other methods.

- Waist-to-Hip Ratio:
  - This is a simple calculation where you measure your waist circumference at its narrowest point and your hip circumference at its widest point. Divide your waist measurement by your hip measurement. A higher ratio may indicate higher body fat.
- Mirror and Visual Estimation:
  - While not as precise, you can visually estimate body fat by comparing your reflection to images of individuals with known body fat percentages. This method is subjective but may give you a general idea.

Remember that these methods provide estimations, and their accuracy can vary. For more accurate results, consider professional methods such as DEXA scans or hydrostatic weighing. Additionally, it's essential to focus on overall health rather than fixating solely on body fat percentage.

Always follow the specific instructions provided with the measurement tool you choose and ensure consistency in your approach to tracking changes over time. If you have any health concerns or conditions, it's advisable to consult with a healthcare provider.

Two Ways to Tell if You Have Too Much Belly Fat

Are you worried that you may have too much belly fat? Here are two simple ways to answer that question.

- *Method One: Waist Circumference*

The Waist-to-Hip Ratio (WHR) is a simple calculation that involves measuring your waist circumference and hip circumference. Here's a step-by-step guide with a detailed example:

Step 1: Gather Tools
- You'll need a flexible measuring tape.

Step 2: Measure Waist Circumference
- Find the narrowest part of your waist, usually just above your belly button.
- Hold the measuring tape snugly around your waist without compressing the skin.
- Ensure the tape is parallel to the ground and is not twisted.
- Record the measurement in inches or centimeters.

Step 3: Measure Hip Circumference
- Locate the widest part of your hips, typically around the hip bones.
- Keep the measuring tape horizontal and wrap it around the fullest part of your hips and buttocks.
- Record the measurement in inches or centimeters.

Step 4: Calculate Waist-to-Hip Ratio
- Divide your waist circumference by your hip circumference.

Example:
- Waist Circumference: 30 inches
- Hip Circumference: 40 inches
- Waist-to-Hip Ratio = Waist Circumference / Hip Circumference
- Waist-to-Hip Ratio = 30 inches / 40 inches
- Waist-to-Hip Ratio = 0.75

In this example, the Waist-to-Hip Ratio is 0.75.

Interpretation:
- WHR values can provide insights into body fat distribution and associated health risks.

Generally:

- For women, a WHR below 0.80 is considered low risk, 0.80-0.85 moderate risk, and above 0.85 high risk.
- For men, a WHR below 0.95 is considered low risk, 0.95-1.0 moderate risk, and above 1.0 high risk.

WHR is just one indicator, and health assessment should consider multiple factors. If you have concerns about your health, it's advisable to consult with a healthcare provider.

According to the Centers for Disease Control and Prevention, having excessive abdominal fat, which is defined as a waist circumference of more than forty inches for a man or more than thirty-five inches for a non-pregnant woman, may place you at increased risk of obesity-related conditions. However, this measure may be inaccurate for people who are shorter than average. A short man or woman may have excessive body fat, even with a waist measurement of less than thirty-five inches for a woman or forty inches for a man. Regardless of this, measuring your waist every month or two can help you determine whether you're losing this dangerous fat.

- *Method Two: Waist-to-Height Ratio*

Step 1: Gather Tools
- You will need a fabric tape.

Step 2: Measure your waist.
- Measure your waist while standing.
- Place a fabric tape measure around your bare stomach and just above the crest of your pelvis or hipbone.
- Make sure that the tape measure is level all around and pull it so that it's snug but not so tight that it causes any sort of bulging.
- Relax and exhale without pushing your stomach out or sucking it in. Just let your stomach sit in its natural state.

Step 3: Calculate Waist-to-Height Ratio
- Convert your height into inches and divide your waist measurement by your height.

That number is your waist-to-height ratio. So, a man who is five feet eight inches tall has a height of sixty-eight inches. If his waist is thirty-four inches, his waist-to-height ratio is 0.50. Ideally, you want a number that's in the healthy range of 0.46 to 0.51. Research suggests that a waist-to-height ratio of .52 or higher puts you at a higher risk of developing obesity-related diseases. Tracking your waist-to-height ratio is another way to determine whether your belly fat is decreasing.

- *The Standard American Diet (SAD)*

You just learned about the dangers of belly fat, so now, let's take a look at the primary cause of belly fat — the standard American diet. Yes, we're not as active as we used to be, so we're expending fewer calories than we used to, but it's really the way we eat that is contributing to excess body fat, particularly belly fat.

While there are exceptions, most of us eat a diet that contains a lot of processed, packaged foods. We consume too many hydrogenated vegetable oils or trans fats. We consume far too much sugar and alcohol. We eat too many simple carbohydrates, many of which contain almost no nutritional value.

At the same time, we fail to eat enough of the foods that fight inflammation: vegetables, fruits, whole grains, and healthy fats. Complicating matters is that the Standard American Diet (SAD) falls short of many important nutrients our bodies need. When we consume our food too quickly or eat in a stressed-out state, which happens frequently, we can't digest food properly, which leads to indigestion and gastrointestinal problems.

It's important to understand the prevalence and attraction of processed foods and carbohydrates. They're inexpensive, readily available, and they taste oh so good, so good, in fact, that we're addicted to them. In particular, sugar and wheat can trigger inflammation not only in the gut but also in the brain. Author, neurologist, and medical expert David Perlmutter MD explains the relationship between the brain and gut in his bestseller book, GRAIN BRAIN, "The Surprising Truth About Wheat, Carbs, Sugar — Your Brain's Silent Killers."

There's a feedback loop between your gut — specifically the microbiota or bacteria living there (called the *microbiome*) — and your brain. When you eat pro-inflammatory food, your gut produces substances that generate an inflammatory reaction. Those substances are carried via your circulatory and nervous system to your brain. They cross the blood-brain barrier and cause inflammation, affecting the neurotransmitters in the brain.

We now know anxiety and depression can be caused by inflammation in the brain and nervous system. We are beginning to realize the powerful connection between the gut, which researchers sometimes call the second brain.

Fortunately, you can affect your gut and your brain with healthy lifestyle choices. In addition to eating anti-inflammatory foods, research suggests that exercise, stress reduction, prayer, and meditation positively impact the microbiome and promote brain health. Many physicians have ignored this connection, but today, there's growing interest in the gut-brain axis, gut-liver axis, gut-skin axis, and their overall impact on health. Despite the increase in conversation about gut health, more research is required in this area as we continue to discover how the gut affects the other areas of the body.

A Brief History of Dietary Recommendations
Have you ever wondered where dietary recommendations come from? When the United States Department of Agriculture's first food guide appeared more than one hundred years ago in 1917, it ignored limiting sugars and fats (In 1902, Wilbur Olin Atwater, PhD., an agricultural chemist

and researcher, published a USDA farmer's bulletin listing healthy foods and advising the limited intake of fat, sugar, and starchy carbohydrates).

After the first Recommended Daily Allowances (RDA) was issued in 1940, the *National Nutrition Guide* in 1946 set out the concept of the four basic food groups (milk, meat, fruits and vegetables, and grain products). Historically, there has been a heavy emphasis on eating grain products (the category in which sugars and carbohydrates belong). This is likely to have been because the secretary of agriculture was pushing for greater consumption of grain products. He recommended six to eleven servings a day.

Several iterations later, including borrowing a model from Sweden's food pyramid in the 1980s, the USDA published its current food pyramid model in 2010. Did the panel of experts take into consideration all the research that supported eating a higher protein, healthy fat, and lower carbohydrate diet? Of course not. This would conflict with the interests of our nation's agricultural department, not to mention the food processing industry. Keep this in mind when you consider the recommendations.

Sugar, the Sweet Poison, and the Reason It's So Deadly

As a country, we are consuming more sugar per person than ever before, and it's having an enormous impact on our health. Some experts go as far as to call it *white death*. From where we stand today, I would have to agree. It's poison.

Authors have been warning Americans about the dangers of sugar since the early seventies, with books like William Dufty's bestselling *Sugar Blues,* which sold millions of copies. Since then, books like the *Sugar Busters* series, *Suicide by Sugar*, and *Sugar Nation* have all broadcast the message that we are a nation that is addicted to sugar.

Sugar is poison. Sugar is literally killing us, and we don't seem to care. The United States continues to be one of the top consumers of sugar (more than most other nations in the world). A 2015 study found that, on average, Americans now consume 126.4 grams (32 teaspoons) of sugar per day. That is nearly 102 pounds of sugar per year per person! This is two-and-a-half times the recommended daily amount. The World Health Organization recommends an average of 50 grams per person per day, so the difference is roughly 2.5 times the recommended amount. The American Heart Association (AHA) has even stricter guidelines for daily added sugar consumption (6 teaspoons or 25 grams) for most women and children (about nine teaspoons or 36 grams) for most men.

Regardless of how our nation is doing in this area, consider your own personal relationship to sugar. Unless they are tested and diagnosed with diabetes, most people have no idea what their blood sugar levels are, how strong their insulin response is, or even what an insulin response means. Most people have no idea how much sugar they're consuming on a daily basis.

Sugar is sneaky because it's in nearly everything; even healthy fruit and vegetable juices contain lots of added sugar. Slugging down eight or ten ounces of juice without the pectin, fiber, and other nutrients that whole fruits and vegetables provide can send your blood sugar soaring.

When you eat sugar, your body releases insulin into your bloodstream to absorb extra sugar or glucose to stabilize sugar levels. Insulin is a hormone made in your pancreas. When you eat too much, over time, your body can develop insulin resistance. This means that it won't respond to sugar when it needs to. Then, the excess sugar ends up being processed by the only other organ that can handle it: the liver.

However, the liver may already be overworked because of all the other foods and chemicals we've dumped into it, so inflammation and disease begin to grow. You won't notice this at first, not until it's too late.

All this leads to metabolic dysfunction, causes weight gain, decreases HDL (good cholesterol), increases LDL (bad cholesterol), elevates triglycerides, and causes high blood pressure. When you overwork your pancreas by requiring it to pump out insulin to combat your addiction for years and years, it will give up. It's now done, kaput. Your pancreas may go on strike and refuse to regularly produce insulin. What is the result? Diabetes.

What's so bad about diabetes? You can just take a pill or an insulin injection, and then you'll be okay, right? Well… maybe. But what typically happens is that people with diabetes struggle to maintain normal blood glucose levels. Blood-glucose levels that are too high damage nerves and blood vessels. That, in turn, increases your risk of developing heart disease and stroke, which are the leading causes of death for people with diabetes.

Your risk doesn't end there. Uncontrolled diabetes can lead to neuropathy (a lack of proper nerve function), kidney failure, vision loss, and limb amputations.

Are Artificial Sweeteners the Solution?
The Short Answer Is No

Are you wondering if artificial sweeteners are a better choice than sugar? They may contain fewer calories, but they're even worse than real sugar because of the way our bodies react to them. In short, they create an insulin response that's even more dramatic than the one sugar produces. They promote weight gain, may increase hunger, and cause metabolic confusion.

They also promote other health problems such as cardiovascular disease, stroke, and Alzheimer's disease. Studies show that avoiding artificial sweeteners like Splenda may help prevent uncomfortable gastrointestinal symptoms. These symptoms result from an overgrowth of E. coli bacteria or other unhealthy bacteria, which, in turn, causes inflammation. Your best bet is to completely avoid artificial sweeteners like aspartame, acesulfame, and saccharin. Some studies suggest that erythritol may contribute to symptoms such as bloating, diarrhea, gas, stomach pain, and nausea. Preliminary research indicates it is associated with an increased risk of heart attack and stroke. It's important to note that further research is needed to comprehensively understand the effects of erythritol on different individuals. Additionally, maltitol, another sugar alcohol, has been associated with gastrointestinal distress at elevated levels.

I've focused a lot on sugar in this section because it's one of the largest dietary contributors to inflammation. However, once you know how to identify the primary sources of sugar in your diet, it's easier to limit it. In Chapter 6, you'll learn how to eat to fight inflammation, which foods to avoid, which foods are natural inflammation reducers, and how to incorporate more of them into your diet. Then, in Chapter 10, you'll learn which supplements help combat inflammation.

Are You Chronically Under-Hydrated? Water's Influence on Inflammation

There's another aspect of your diet that can influence how inflamed you are: how much or how little water you drink. The bottom line is that many of us fail to drink enough water, which leads to chronic dehydration. You'll learn about how to estimate your body's needs and how to drink more water in Chapter 6. For now, let's look at what happens when you're under-hydrated and the reason that this makes inflammation worse.

Water is an essential part of every cell in your body. Your blood cells need fluid to flow. Your heart, which is a giant muscle, needs fluid to beat. Your body needs a way to flush out all the intracellular waste that clogs up its lymphatic system.

Underhydration happens when you consume less water than your body needs or when your body loses large amounts of fluids and salts. Your body then lacks enough fluid to function normally. When you lose as little as one percent of your total water volume, you'll begin to experience symptoms of under-hydration, which include mood changes, a lowered ability to concentrate, fatigue, increased perception of task difficulty, and headaches. You're also unable to flush out toxins efficiently.

Do you think thirst is a good indicator of whether you're under-hydrated or not? Think again. If you feel thirsty, it's already too late. You're officially at least 2 percent dehydrated. If you lose even more water, you may experience the following: headaches, migraines, dizziness, weakness, extreme fatigue, dry skin, dry mouth and lips, irritability, depression, inability to concentrate, inability to perform regular daily tasks, loss of energy, lower level of consciousness, constipation, muscle cramps, joint pain, and back pain. Your immune system becomes compromised, and you're more prone to catching a cold or the flu.

When moderate to severe dehydration occurs, you may experience fainting, convulsions, low blood pressure, severe muscle cramping, heart failure, dry eyes, wrinkled skin (because of loss of elasticity), rapid breathing, a fast and weak pulse, and a bloated abdomen. In cases of severe dehydration, the above symptoms worsen, your pulse and blood pressure may become undetectable, your skin may become pale, and ultimately, death may occur. But even milder dehydration, if chronic, can lead to kidney stones and affect kidney function as well. It can also lead to muscle damage, including damage to the heart.

In many cases, instead of taking an antacid (more chemicals for your body to process), drinking water will help reduce or eliminate problems with indigestion or heartburn. While water on its own doesn't overcome inflammation, sufficient water is an essential element in how your body fights it. What is the takeaway? Chronic underhydration can be a factor in chronic inflammation.

- *Stress*

As a society, we're stressed out. According to a recent poll by Gallup, four out of ten adults feel stress sometimes or frequently throughout their day. The American Psychological Association, which conducts an annual *Stress in America* survey, has found that Americans' stress levels have increased in the last several years.

While you often hear people complain about being stressed or feel it yourself, you may not really understand what stress means when it comes to your body's response to it and the way that it impacts inflammation. Your body experiences two main types of stress: psychological stress (mental and emotional) and physical stress.

Physical stress refers to things that challenge your body, such as healing from an injury or exercising. It is anything that taxes your body's resources. Physical stress is easy to identify. Unless you're worn out or run down, your body is generally able to handle it.

Psychological stress includes the stress that is caused by emotions and mental pressure. When you experience psychological stress, your body pumps more cortisol and other stress hormones into your system, which contributes to inflammation.

In order to fully understand its impact, let's look at what might happen to someone on a typical day. First, stressors are introduced. Usually, there's more than one on any given day. Some scenarios might be that traffic causes you to arrive late to a meeting, a child wakes up sick, you wake up sick, you have too many deadlines, your work is unorganized, you have too many bills, your spouse is upset about the bills, or your spouse wants a divorce. Possibly, dinner is burning on the stove, a loved one dies, your friend is upset that you've been too busy to spend time with them, or you have to move to a new home. Maybe a check bounces, and you are charged extra fees for insufficient funds.

In addition, you change jobs, you fail a test, nobody laughs at your joke, your car stalls, your car needs expensive repairs, and you have to take public transportation in the meantime. This adds time to your already long commute. Perhaps you've gained ten pounds, your in-laws want to visit, your request for vacation was denied, your house is a mess, and you can't find a place to sit in peace.

Do you feel the weight of all of that? That's a lot, and hopefully, you aren't dealing with the entire list at the same time. But many people are. They may feel sad, hopeless, disorganized, pressured, confused, lonely, inadequate, unloved, unappreciated, or a combination of these emotions.

These feelings, in turn, lead to psychological stress and hormonal responses that cause the adrenal glands (each one is located on top of a kidney) to release a surge of cortisol to race through the body. Cortisol inhibits insulin production and constricts the arteries, while its hormonal partner in crime, epinephrine, increases the heart rate. It's the main ingredient of your fight-or-flight response.

Now, your heart is pumping harder and faster. If you have any plaque buildup in your arteries from the fatty processed foods you've been eating, you're a prime candidate for heart disease and a stroke. Your immune system is weakened. Digestion comes to a halt. Blood sugar rises.

Stress also manifests itself in other places in the body. Having a tight jaw or grinding your teeth can lead to dental issues or, worse, temporal mandibular joint (TMJ) pain. Tightness in shoulders and knots in muscles like the trapezius and rhomboids lead to neck and back issues. Stress causes headaches, migraines, ulcers, fatigue, depression, diabetes, cancer, panic attacks, and immune deficiency.

Before we completely demonize cortisol, I should tell you that cortisol itself isn't all bad. In fact, it's there to protect us. In addition to helping manage blood pressure, it's actually meant to help fight stress, and it converts protein into fuel during a perceived stressful event. The key here is that cortisol responds to threats, whether they are real or not.

We're no longer living among wild animals where we need the fight-or-flight response. There are occasions when people face imminent life-threatening danger, but those are usually very rare. Yet our bodies, which are controlled by our minds, act as if everyday life poses life-threatening situations. We need to retrain the body-mind connection so that we can recognize the difference between real threats and perceived threats.

Chronic stress can have the same effects and can be caused by a stressful, demanding job, a demanding boss, children who continually misbehave, toxic dead-end relationships, a messy, unorganized home or office, watching the nightly news, a nosy neighbor, or simply reading a continuous flow of negative posts on social media.

You can experience all kinds of stressful scenarios yet not be affected by them. How do you do this? You do this by becoming aware of it. Change your perception of events so that they are different from what you may have earlier considered stressful. Once your brain no longer perceives a threatening event or resolves the situation, your cortisol levels return to normal. It stays that way unless the stress response is triggered again.

With the *Extinguish the Flame Program*, you'll learn how to reduce the number of stressors you have in your life and the impact of stressors you can't avoid. In Chapter 8, you'll learn the importance of play, laughter, love, and gratitude and how to incorporate more of these things into your life.

- *Lack of Quality Sleep*

As I pointed out earlier in this chapter, some of these inflammatory factors interrelate with each other. With so many people complaining of occasional or frequent stress, it's not surprising that a number of us have trouble sleeping as well. It is estimated that about one-third of all adults experience insomnia (trouble falling asleep or staying asleep) on a regular basis. Between fifty and seventy million people have a sleep disorder.

Various data have shown that the average person sleeps only seven hours a night. More than one-third of these people say that they sleep less than that. So it doesn't come as a complete shock that four in ten of us have admitted to falling asleep during the day at least once in the last month.

While it's normal to experience a bad night's sleep occasionally, if it occurs regularly, you're setting yourself up for problems. Deep sleep is what fuels our daily activities. Insomnia can starve your body of what it needs to sustain you during your waking hours.

According to Healthline, at least seven hours of sleep is the recommended amount for most adults. However, it is more about the quality of sleep that you get. I've found that quality usually depends on many factors, including diet and, you guessed it, inflammation. People who have restless sleep often wake up several times throughout the night and never get into that deep rapid-eye-movement (REM) sleep. REM sleep is important because it is the restorative part of your sleep cycle and stimulates the regions of the brain that are used in learning and memory.

The causes of sleeplessness are multifactorial. People are undernourished and over-caffeinated. Caffeine is perhaps the biggest culprit of sleepless nights. Many of us are connected to screens of some sort (televisions, computers, electronic tablets, and smartphones) up to the time we go to bed. The light from these screens tricks our brains into thinking it's daytime. A lack of exercise and a lack of other stress-busting techniques also contribute to the problem.

Those factors affect sleep quality, but sometimes, we *choose* to sacrifice sleep for other things. Going into nocturnal overdrive to get a job done or to hang out with friends may seem harmless, but you could be sacrificing your health if you do it regularly. Your body doesn't know that you wanted to celebrate your friend's birthday. It recognizes your lack of sleep as a state of stress.

As you saw earlier in this chapter, once you are in stress mode, your body responds by raising the levels of stress hormones such as adrenaline and cortisol. Hormones regulate functions such as blood pressure and insulin levels. When you are in a constant state of stress, these levels can be difficult to control. Your immune system becomes impaired, and then your ability to fight diseases drops.

You should consider sleep a necessity and not a luxury. Even mild sleep deprivation disrupts the normal levels of the hormone's ghrelin and leptin, which regulate appetite. Low levels of leptin can make you crave carbs and overeat. Studies show that those who sleep less are more prone to gain weight than those who spend more time asleep.

Are you still not convinced of sleep's importance? Take a look at the physiological effects of sleep deprivation.

- blurry vision
- cognitive impairment, memory lapses, and mental inefficiency
- dark under-eye circles
- depression
- fatigue
- hallucinations and psychosis
- headaches
- heart palpitations
- hyperactivity
- irritability
- impaired immune system
- increased blood pressure
- irritability
- muscle aches
- weight gain, or less frequently, weight loss

Usually, the symptoms of short-term sleep deprivation can be reversed by getting the proper amount of sleep right away. However, long-term sleep deprivation contributes to inflammation. In Chapter 9, you'll learn how to set the stage for restful quality sleep.

How Inflammation Factors Impact You

In this chapter, you've learned more about the primary factors causing inflammation and the reason that they're so dangerous. In the next chapter, you'll have a chance to personalize this information. Read on to determine which of these factors are affecting you.

Chapter 3
How Inflamed Are You?

Getting a Sense of the Problem

The vast preponderance of evidence in modern epidemiology shows that those who eat more whole plant foods and fewer animal products and processed foods have lower rates of chronic disease and longer lifespans.

- Joel Fuhrman, MD, physician and author

In the last chapter, you learned about the primary factors that trigger inflammation and how prevalent they are. It's possible and even likely that your body has been dealing with chronic inflammation for years or decades, even if you're not currently experiencing symptoms. Maybe you do have symptoms but haven't attributed them to inflammation.

This chapter is designed to help you identify how much inflammation you may have. Even more importantly, you can review these factors at any time (like after you make the lifestyle changes suggested by the *Extinguish the Flame Program*) to see how much you've reduced your risk of inflammation. If you want an even more detailed analysis, in the next chapter, you'll learn about the lab tests you can take to measure different markers of inflammation.

Your Exposure to Environmental Factors

First, let's look at the environmental factors you're exposed to. Answer each statement with one of the following: constantly, frequently, occasionally, or rarely/never. Give yourself four points for each constant answer, three points for each frequently, two points for each occasionally, and one point for each rarely/never. Write that number down next to the statement.

- I use pesticides and/or herbicides in my yard or garden.
- I use household cleansers.
- I wear perfume or cologne.
- I wear deodorant or antiperspirant that contains aluminum and/or parabens (Unless the product says "paraben-free" on the label, it probably contains parabens).
- I use beauty products (like soap and shampoo) that contain parabens.
- I work in buildings that contain formaldehyde (Many buildings are constructed using this chemical, which is a known carcinogen or cause of cancer).
- I live in a city or area where the air quality is poor.
- I walk near heavily trafficked areas, and I am exposed to exhaust fumes.
- I smoke, or I am exposed to secondhand smoke.
- I take over-the-counter or prescription medication for digestive problems, pain, high blood pressure, high cholesterol, depression, or anxiety.

Now, add up your total score and write it below.

Environmental Toxins Score: ____

Physical and Emotional Symptoms of Inflammation
Next, consider the physical and emotional symptoms of inflammation that you may have. Answer each statement with one of the following: constantly, frequently, occasionally, or rarely/never. Give yourself four points for each constant answer, three points for each frequently, two points for each occasionally, and one point for each rarely/never. Write that number down next to the statement (except for the one about pinching an inch).

- I have headaches and/or migraines.

- I have chronic aches and pains (like neck or back soreness or joint pain).
- I have heartburn or digestive issues like an upset stomach, gas, or bloating.
- I suffer from allergies, colds, or flu symptoms.
- I can grab at least an inch of extra fat around my waist (Give yourself four points if you can, and one point if you cannot).
- I feel tired throughout the day.
- I feel mentally lethargic or have a tough time focusing.
- I feel depressed or sad for no apparent reason.
- I have insomnia or trouble sleeping.
- I have one or more of the following conditions: arthritis, fibromyalgia, chronic fatigue syndrome, sinusitis, allergies, acne, asthma, dysmenorrhea (menstrual pain/cramps), endometriosis, Alzheimer's disease, Parkinson's disease, multiple sclerosis, cancer, heart disease, osteoporosis, hypertension, depression, insulin resistance syndrome (prediabetes), or diabetes (Give yourself four points for each condition that you have).

Now, add up your total score and write it below.

Physical and Emotional Symptoms Score: _____

Negative Dietary and Lifestyle Factors
Your diet and lifestyle have powerful impacts on whether you have inflammation. Answer each statement with one of the following: constantly, frequently, occasionally, or rarely/never. Give yourself four points for each constant answer, three points for each frequently, two points for each occasionally, and one point for each rarely/never. Write that number down next to the statement.

- I eat grains and grain products such as white bread, whole wheat bread, pasta, cereal, pretzels, crackers, and any other product made with grains or flour from

grains (which includes most desserts and packaged snacks).
- I eat refined sugar in things like desserts, cookies, candy, soda, or other sweetened beverages.
- I consume fried foods or packaged foods (both are sources of partially hydrogenated oils or trans fats).
- I consume margarine and/or oils like corn oil, safflower oil, sunflower oil, cottonseed oil, or soybean oil (including foods made with them like mayonnaise, tartar sauce, and nearly all salad dressings).
- I consume fewer than nine servings of fruits and vegetables a day.
- I eat meat and eggs from grain-fed animals (which include most of the brands you find at the supermarket).
- I drink alcohol.
- The quality of my sleep is poor, or I sleep fewer than seven hours a night.
- I don't exercise.
- I have little time to spend with the people that I enjoy.

Now, add up your total score and write it below.

Negative Dietary and Lifestyle Factors Score: _____

Positive Dietary and Lifestyle Factors

Fortunately, you may already be doing some things that help reverse inflammation. Answer each statement with one of the following: constantly, frequently, occasionally, and rarely/never. Give yourself four points for each constant answer, three points for each frequently, two points for each occasionally, and one point for each rarely/never. Write that number down next to the statement.

- I eat at least nine servings of vegetables and fruit every day.
- I consume olive oil or other heart-healthy oils.
- I consume fatty fish (like tuna, salmon, and sardines).

- I consume whole-grain foods (if you're not gluten-sensitive).
- I avoid junk food and sugary foods whenever I can.
- I take breaks during my workday.
- I make an effort to move throughout my day.
- I meditate, pray, or take time to consider the things I'm grateful for.
- I spend time with friends or family members who make me laugh.
- I have hobbies that I enjoy.

Now, add up your total score and write it below.

Positive Dietary and Lifestyle Factors ____

Add it Up: Your Extinguish the Flame Inflammation Score

To get your total inflammation score, add up the first three totaled sums and then subtract the Positive Dietary and Lifestyle Factor score from it. If your score is less than twenty, congratulations! It appears that you're in the clear as far as inflammation goes.

Maintaining the healthy lifestyle that the *Extinguish the Flame Program* sets out will help you continue to fight it. If your score is twenty-one to forty, you likely have some degree of inflammation. The *Extinguish the Flame Program* will help decrease it.

If your score is more than forty-one, you're likely suffering from significant inflammation and should take immediate action to reverse it before you have a major health crisis. Are you frightened by your score? Keep in mind that even small positive steps in the right direction can help you fight inflammation and make you healthier, both now and in the future.

So don't be overwhelmed by factors that you can't change, such as if you live in an urban environment with poor air quality. Focus on the changes you *can* make.

This chapter gave you a sense of the degree of inflammation you may have by looking at varied factors contributing to it. In the next chapter, we'll look inside your body and find out what happens when inflammation takes hold.

Chapter 4
From the Inside Out

How Inflammation Affects Your Body

At the end of the day, your health is your responsibility.

- Jillian Michaels, fitness expert

It's tempting to put your health in the hands of others — your doctor's or even your spouse's. But your body is *your* responsibility and not your doctor's or your mate's. You alone are responsible for what you put into it and on it. You are responsible for learning how it functions and knowing how it works. You are the only one with the power to contribute to its health or to its demise.

In the last chapter, you got a sense of how inflamed you may be, but let's dig deeper and look at what's happening inside your body. In this chapter, you'll learn about a few of your body's critical organs and their functions, as well as how you can have the greatest impact by making lifestyle changes like the ones in the *Extinguish the Flame Program*.

What's My Score? Tests That Help Measure Inflammation

Before we discuss certain laboratory tests that measure inflammation, let's consider how to determine what's happening inside your body. While this book isn't about all of the nuances of Western medicine, it is about raising awareness. If knowing is half the battle to achieving anything (including your best possible health), there's really only one way to find out what your actual state of health is: by testing. This is what qualified health professionals do best. You may feel great, but there could be some silent disease lurking inside you that testing may help reveal before it becomes catastrophic.

You may already receive a complete metabolic and lipid panel at your annual checkup. This blood test measures blood glucose and total cholesterol, including HDL (good) and LDL (bad) cholesterol. It also measures the levels of minerals in your body, including calcium, iron, and potassium. If you have diabetes or if your doctor suspects you might, you'll probably also have your hemoglobin A1C checked, which determines your blood sugar levels over the previous months.

While there are numerous methods for measuring inflammation, these tests are just a start. Talk to your healthcare provider about the tests that are right for you and discuss the results with them.

- *C-Reactive Protein and High-Sensitivity-CRP (hs-CRP)*

C-reactive protein is one of the most widely known indicators of inflammation. A simple blood test measures how much of it is in your body. Hs-CRP is more sensitive than regular C-reactive protein and may catch inflammation much earlier.

- *Ferritin*

This blood test tends to be more elevated with chronic or long-standing inflammation. It can also mean your body is storing too much iron (iron overload).

- *Cortisol/DHEA*

This simple saliva or blood test measures levels of the stress hormone cortisol, a marker for adrenal fatigue, and dehydroepiandrosterone (DHEA), which is often referred to as the anti-aging hormone produced by the adrenal glands.

- *Vitamin D3*

About one in three adults is deficient in vitamin D. However, if you take supplements, you can consume too much of this vitamin. Monitoring your vitamin D level is especially helpful if you're dealing with problems like bone weakness and malformation or abnormal metabolism of calcium.

- *Homocysteine*

A blood test will check your levels of homocysteine, an amino acid associated with inflammation and an increased risk of heart disease.

- *Food Sensitivity*

These tests measure your body's immune response to specific foods to help determine whether you're allergic or sensitive to any of them.

- *Neurotransmitter Analysis*

This is usually a urine test. It measures your levels of neurotransmitters like serotonin. Levels of neurotransmitters that are too high or too low contribute to hormone imbalances, depression, anxiety, and weight gain.

- *Omega-3 Test*

This blood test helps determine the levels of omega-3 fatty acids in your blood. It is an indicator of your risk for cardiovascular disease.

- *Prostate-Specific Antigen Test (PSA) and Prostate Health Index Test (PHI)*

For men only, this test measures possible inflammation in the prostate gland. The prostate health index (PHI) is one such test that is a more accurate blood test and measures your risk for having prostate cancer. It's approved by the FDA for men who have PSA scores between 4 and 10.

- *Sleep Apnea Test*

Undiagnosed sleep apnea is a leading cause of poor-quality sleep. This test, which is usually performed overnight in a sleep lab, helps determine whether you have a sleep disorder.

- *Micronutrient Test*

This blood test measures levels of different micronutrients, which can help you determine whether you have a specific nutrient deficiency.

- *Microbiome Test*

This test examines the composition of microorganisms in your digestive system, known as the gut microbiome. These microorganisms play a vital role in various bodily functions, including digestion, immune system regulation, and even influencing mood. By assessing the diversity and balance of bacteria in your gut, a microbiome test can help identify potential imbalances that may contribute to inflammation and other health issues.

- *Testosterone or Estradiol*

These blood tests can help determine whether your sex hormones are at healthy levels. For example, low levels of testosterone are linked with abdominal obesity and inflammation.

- *Full Thyroid Panel*

This test provides a comprehensive view of thyroid function. An imbalance of any tests within the panel may be associated with inflammation.

While there are other tests available for determining inflammation, we have listed some of the most popular.

The Interplay of Your Body's Organs and Systems

Taking some of the just-mentioned tests can give you a peek inside your body. When it comes to your body, no organ functions on its own. Your body is a closed system. Just as your gut health affects your brain's health, every organ and system affects the others. This is the reason why local inflammation can quickly become more widespread. Even a minor inflammatory event that is left unchecked can progress to other parts of your body. Read on to learn more about some of your body's amazing organs and the ways that they help keep you healthy.

- *The Liver: The Detoxifier*

My personal favorite organ is the liver, which is perhaps the most underrated and misunderstood organ in the body. It is nothing short of a powerhouse. The liver works nonstop to process everything you consume and detoxify your body. This includes everything that you inhale, swallow, or absorb into your skin.

The liver's function is to cleanse the blood, regulate the supply of fuel, blood sugar, and cholesterol, support calcium absorption, convert vitamin D, and manufacture essential body proteins. It also produces bile, which not only aids in digestion but is also the primary way your body eliminates toxic substances. The liver is the largest organ, second to our skin. It performs more than five hundred functions and is the only organ that can regenerate itself. At any given time, it contains about 10 percent of the body's blood supply.

The liver works hard, but you may force it to work harder than it should. Consider what you eat and drink on a regular basis. If, like most people, you are eating something similar to the Standard American Diet, your diet is laden with processed foods with ingredients that you can't even pronounce. Your liver must detoxify these chemicals. That includes alcohol, sugary juices, soda, refined sugar, enriched flour, artificial flavorings, processed and fatty meats, unhealthy oils (including hydrogenated and trans fats), fillers, preservatives, drugs (both prescription and recreational), and toxins from intestinal microbes. The average person's liver is overworked, and it is choking on the poisons that we're feeding it.

Alcohol has long been a known nemesis to the liver, but doctors are slowly becoming more aware of the impact refined sugar is having on liver function as well. A diet high in simple sugars can lead to fat building up in the liver as well, which then leads to inflammation and scar tissue. *Fatty liver* refers to what happens when the liver has fatty buildup. This can progress through several stages to non-alcoholic steatohepatitis (NASH), which causes cirrhosis of the liver and liver cancer. In fact, NASH is a growing reason for liver transplants. In addition to avoiding as many toxins as possible, slashing your daily sugar intake can have a dramatic impact on your liver's function.

It's also crucial to be aware of non-alcoholic fatty liver disease (NAFLD), a condition characterized by excessive fat accumulation in the liver unrelated to alcohol consumption. NAFLD encompasses a spectrum of liver conditions, ranging from simple fatty liver (steatosis) to (NASH). NAFLD is closely linked to lifestyle factors, including diet, obesity, and sedentary behavior. Addressing sugar intake and adopting a liver-friendly lifestyle can play an essential role in preventing and managing NAFLD and promoting overall liver health.

- *The Lungs: Your Body's Bellows*

Your lungs are the largest organ in your respiratory system. Just as your liver filters everything that you eat and drink, your lungs filter the air that you breathe. In the lungs, oxygen is picked up by red blood cells and is carried throughout your body so that any toxins you inhale can be transported throughout your body. As you read earlier, they are ultimately filtered by your liver.

Smoking and secondhand smoke have the biggest impact on your lungs, with air pollution next in line. When you inhale smoke, you are taking in dozens of noxious chemicals that interfere with air filtration. This causes an overproduction of mucus and paralyzes the tiny hair-like cilia in the lungs, which clean out dust and particles. This chain of events leads to inflamed air passages and, ultimately, to smokers' coughs.

For optimal lung function, reduce your exposure to as many airborne toxins as possible. You'll learn more about how to do this in the next chapter. If you smoke, quit and avoid exposure to secondhand smoke and other lung irritants.

- *The Pancreas: Converter of Food into Energy*

Your pancreas is part of the digestive system. It converts the food you eat into fuel for your body's cells. It produces insulin, which regulates blood sugar. If your pancreas can no longer produce insulin, you will develop diabetes.

Several major blood vessels surround the pancreas and supply it with blood. If your blood is carrying too many toxins, which your overburdened liver wasn't able to filter, they can build up here and lead to inflammation and pancreatitis. Left untreated, you can develop pancreatic cancer.

While the exact cause of pancreatic cancer is unknown, research suggests cigarette smoking, chronic pancreatitis, and a family history of pancreatic cancer are factors in determining how likely you are to develop it. Avoiding toxins and eating anti-inflammatory foods will help your pancreas function optimally.

- *The Heart: The Vital Pump*

Your heart is part of your circulatory system. It pumps blood to the lungs and through all the systems of the body. However, plaque buildup in the arteries can lead to cardiovascular disease and ultimately to a heart attack or a stroke. Plaque is caused by a buildup of bad cholesterol, calcium, and other chemicals, as they bind together and stick anywhere they can. It eventually hardens (which is where the phrase hardening of the arteries comes from) and narrows your blood vessels.

Your body responds to this buildup with inflammation, as it perceives the plaque as something foreign that must be removed. Here's where it gets even worse. That inflammation, in turn, may make plaque worse, triggering even more inflammation.

In addition, each cell in every tissue of your body needs a healthy supply of clean blood in order to function properly. If your heart isn't strong enough to pump blood to all parts of the body, any neglected tissue will die. Regular activity, which gets your blood flowing, is crucial to maintaining healthy blood flow. Exercise, along with a healthy diet, also helps prevent plaque buildup and increases good cholesterol, which helps transport bad cholesterol out of the body.

- *The Kidneys: Filtration Machines*

Your kidneys are responsible for filtering your blood. In the process, they remove waste and excess water (the urine that is stored in your bladder). Your kidneys also produce hormones and remove acid from your body, which helps maintain a healthy balance of minerals, salts, and water.

When your kidneys become inflamed, however, it's harder for them to filter blood the way they should. Over time, this can develop into chronic kidney disease, which means that your kidneys are damaged and that the waste they would normally remove can build up in your body.

One of the simplest ways to help your kidneys function well is to drink plenty of water (You'll learn more about this in Chapter 6). In addition, maintaining a healthy body weight, being active, cutting back on salt, and limiting alcohol will also help your kidneys work properly.

- *The Gallbladder: Digestive Helper*

Your gallbladder is a small organ located under your liver. It stores and concentrates the bile produced by the liver so that the small intestine can digest and absorb fat more efficiently.

When your gallbladder is inflamed, you may be more likely to develop gallstones, hardened deposits of cholesterol, or pigment that can be as small as a grain of sand or as large as a golf ball. We don't know the exact cause of gallstones, but factors increasing your risk of developing them are also associated with inflammation. For example, people who are sedentary, eat a diet high in unhealthy fats (like the Standard American Diet), and are overweight or obese are more likely to develop gallstones.

They can also lead to a condition called cholecystitis, which happens when a gallstone becomes stuck in the neck of the gallbladder. Gallstones can also block the bile duct or pancreatic duct, causing pain and infection.

There is one good thing: You can live without a gallbladder. But why should you? Maintaining a healthy body weight and consuming a diet that includes healthy fats and is low in sugar and refined/processed carbohydrates will also help your gallbladder function at its best.

- *Your Gut: Your Body's Second Brain*

You learned in Chapter 2 that the gut is sometimes referred to as your body's second brain. It includes the small and large intestine, which are part of your body's digestive system. This system houses gut bacteria (also called gut flora or microbiome), which helps break down nutrients into smaller parts that your body can use for energy. When your gut is healthy, that process is seamless. When your gut is inflamed, however, pieces of undigested food can leak through the walls of your intestine, triggering even more inflammation and a condition called leaky gut.

If you've ever had an upset stomach after a demanding day, you already know that stress impacts your digestive health. In addition to consuming a diet that is free of gut irritants and includes healthy nutrients, prebiotics, probiotics, postbiotics, butyrate, fiber, adequate hydration, and stress management techniques can help you maintain healthy gut flora and reduce inflammation. Moderate exercise and quality sleep also help keep your gut running smoothly.

- *Your Skin: First Line of Defense against Bacteria and Other Organisms*

The skin is considered the largest organ in the body. It is vital for maintaining overall health and well-being. The skin acts as a barrier against harmful microorganisms, UV radiation, chemicals, and physical injury. It helps prevent dehydration and regulates body temperature. Waste products such as sweat and sebum are excreted through the skin. The skin synthesizes vitamin D from the sun, which plays a role in bone health, brain health, and immune support.

- *Your Brain: Your Body's Command Center*

The brain is your body's computer and the main organ of your central nervous system. It is responsible for communicating messages to all of your systems and organs so that they function properly. When one message is miscommunicated, it can create an entire cascade of mixed and missed messages. You can spend years trying to get the communications back on track.

Two of the biggest influences that impact brain function today are overconsumption of refined sugar and dehydration. Sugar affects our cognitive function and the feedback loop from our brains to our bodies (as you saw in Chapter 2). It's linked to a greater risk of depression and anxiety, it is a leading suspect in dementia, and it is the number one cause of obesity.

As for under-hydration, if you are under-hydrated, even one percent, you lose energy and focus, and your mood will be greatly impacted for the worse. Learning and memory suffer greatly when your brain doesn't have enough water to function. Alertness also diminishes, which can lead to clumsiness and accidents.

When the brain becomes inflamed, it throws off the delicate, healthy balance of neurotransmitters and hormones. Researchers are now exploring the link between inflammation in the brain and conditions like Alzheimer's, Parkinson's, depression, anxiety, attention deficit disorder, and attention deficit hyperactivity disorder. They believe that inflammation may be the root cause of certain mental illnesses as well.

How can you help your brain? You can do this by cutting added sugar from your diet and drinking plenty of water to maintain optimal hydration. Increasing your water intake can also help you maintain healthier eating habits, as thirst often masquerades as hunger. When you're hungry, high-sugar snacks are hard to resist. Equally important are the steps you take to combat inflammation. They will help ensure that the brain's healthy balance of neurotransmitters and other chemicals is maintained.

- *The Big Picture: Your Body as a Whole*

Why should you take time to look more closely at some of your body's organs? What does this have to do with inflammation? Well, your body is a system that has to work as a whole. You may be one organism, but much like members of a small family living in one apartment unit, each organ plays its own role within your body.

Sometimes, we are concerned only with our stomachs or sex organs because we are more aware of their signals. All of our organs have needs. When we embrace a healthy lifestyle, all of our organs and systems will work in harmony. That's the overall goal of the *Extinguish the Flame Program*. In the next six chapters, we'll learn more about what it includes.

Chapter 5
Avoid Pollutants

Step One of the Extinguish the Flame Program

Living healthy in a toxic world...that is the challenge before us.

- author unknown

You now have a more in-depth understanding of what common inflammation is, the damage it can do to your body and overall health, and some of its primary causes. You may feel overwhelmed at this point. Maybe you even think, *Well, what can I do about it?*

Fortunately, the answer is a lot. The six steps of the *Extinguish the Flame Program* don't have to be performed in any particular order, but all of them will help you reduce and combat inflammation. Making small improvements in these different areas can have a significant impact on your health.

There's another important factor here. Consider the psychological factor of knowing that you're doing something healthy for your body. When you choose to eliminate toxins and nurture your body with good stuff, whether that's eating a more nutritious diet, getting better quality sleep, or taking inflammation-fighting supplements, you know you're moving in the right direction. Those steps send the message to your body's organs and cells to begin healing. The power of the mind-body connection cannot be underestimated, especially when it comes to how you think and act about your health.

Reduce Your Exposure to Pollutants and Toxins
In the last chapter, you learned that the more toxins you're exposed to, the harder your liver has to work to process and eliminate them from your body. Now that you realize the impact these kinds of chemicals can have on your body, you'll want to avoid them or reduce your exposure to them whenever possible.

- *Avoid Smoking and Secondhand Smoke*

This is one of the simplest steps you can take to avoid environmental toxins. If you smoke, quit. Smoking is one of the most common causes of inflammation, leading to a multitude of diseases and, eventually, death. (Check out https://smokefree.gov/tools-tips/get-extra-help/free-resources for free tools to help you). Avoid secondhand smoke whenever possible, especially in confined spaces.

- *Breathe Better-Quality Air*

How's the air quality where you live? Do you know? You can visit https://waqi.info to identify your city's air quality index (AQI) in real-time. If the air in your city is regularly low quality and you're able to relocate, you may want to consider doing so. It's also smart to monitor your city's allergen and pollen forecast and avoid going outside during high pollen counts, especially if you have allergies.

At home and at the office, the best type of indoor air protection is an active air purifier. These machines incurporate technology developed by NASA for space travel. Active air purifiers use a unique, new indoor air-quality process to naturally produce airborne scrubbers that actively see out and destroy pollutants, viruses, bacteria, mold, pet dander, pollen, and dust. They also eliminate odors.

These machines differ from normal passive-air or HEPA-filter purifiers, which are inefficient and rely on contaminants floating through the air to find their way to the filtration unit. Passive air systems can only work properly when all the air in the environment physically passes through its mechanical filters so that contaminants can become trapped. Look for air purifiers that utilize multiple technologies to purify your air at home or the office.

Have your gas pipes checked every few years and loose fittings replaced. You probably already have a smoke/carbon-monoxide detector, but you can also purchase an air-quality detector for your home (The air inside your home can contain more toxins than outside air!).

For better air quality indoors, bring air-purifying plants and herbs inside. Instead of using artificial air fresheners, use natural ones like citrus peels, essential oils, or fresh herbs. Take your shoes off at the front door to reduce tracking in bacteria, toxins, and grime (Your floors will stay much cleaner, too).

- *Choose Nontoxic Products*

Many toiletries include chemicals, including parabens, which are known to cause inflammation. In fact, the average woman is exposed to eighteen different chemicals through her beauty products, and the average man is exposed to six different chemicals every day! Look for "parabens and aluminum-free" on the label of products like toothpaste, shampoos, soaps, deodorants, lotions, and cosmetics you buy.

Consider what reasonable changes you can make in your everyday life. For example, paper products like facial tissue, napkins, and paper towels may contain cancer-causing chemicals, so you might swap out paper napkins for all-natural, 100-percent cotton ones. Maybe you use rags instead of paper towels. Obviously, some changes are more convenient than others, so keep in mind that every small step you take, like choosing a natural bug-repellent instead of a chemical-laden one, can add up over time.

One relatively simple change you can make is to opt for nontoxic cleaning products. Read the section titled "Choose Less Toxic Cleaning Supplies." You can reduce dust levels with damp-cleaning methods (a cotton cloth dampened with water) instead of cleaners with heavy toxic chemicals. When buying products for your home, choose cotton and natural fibers over polyester or other man-made fibers.

- *Reduce the Number of Chemicals You Eat and Drink*

Choose fresh organic produce when possible, especially with foods that are likely to otherwise contain pesticides. The Environmental Working Group creates an annual *Dirty Dozen* list of the fruits and vegetables most likely to contain pesticides. In 2018, that list included strawberries, spinach, nectarines, apples, grapes, peaches, cherries, pears, tomatoes, celery, potatoes, and sweet bell peppers. Its *Clean Fifteen* for 2018 included avocadoes, sweet corn, pineapples, cabbages, onions, frozen sweet peas, papayas, asparagus, mangoes, eggplants, honeydews, kiwis, cantaloupes, cauliflower, and broccoli. These are the produce least likely to contain pesticides.

Instead of buying water in plastic bottles for home use, use a water-filtration system. Keep your food in glass and other eco-friendly containers instead of plastic ones.

- *Avoid Yard Chemicals*

Do you grow a garden every summer? Opt for all-natural, chemical-free options to eliminate garden pests and avoid using lawn-care chemicals. You may even want to consider joining the movement Food Not Lawns, where homeowners use their yards to grow produce instead of grass.

- *Avoid Inflammatory-Causing Medications when Possible*

There's one other source of toxins that you may be ingesting without realizing the damaging effects: medications. I believe that the doctors who prescribe these medications think they're helping their patients, but in many cases, they're not. Not only do they fail to dig deeper in order to get to the root of their patient's health problems and educate them about the changes they can make to heal and prevent disease, but some of the medications they prescribe are also harming their patients.

There are plenty of statistics about America's over-reliance on drugs, but the fact is that we use the Band-Aid approach, treating many of our symptoms with drugs. Some anti-inflammatory medications are prescribed to help people with disease, yet the drugs themselves are inflammatory and ultimately cause even more inflammation in the long run.

There are times when an anti-inflammatory drug is necessary for a short time, but we've been programmed to blindly trust our doctors without doing any research on our own, being advocates for ourselves, and considering whether there are holistic alternatives to taking a drug. Many of the drugs that we use today produce side effects that are worse than the actual condition they're designed to treat!

The takeaway isn't to avoid all medications because some of them are necessary. Instead of just filling a prescription because your doctor has suggested it, talk to him or her about its impact on your body and whether there are alternatives and changes you can make to treat your condition without drugs. At the least, you'll be a more informed patient and less likely to take medications you may not even need.

Choose Less Toxic Cleaning Supplies

Until reading this book, you may not have thought about the household cleaners and other products you use at home, but they are often laden with harmful, pro-inflammatory chemicals. According to the American Lung Association, you can reduce your risk of health problems by limiting your exposure to these kinds of chemicals.

First, read the labels and follow the instructions carefully. For example, some products are flammable or shouldn't be used without good ventilation. Keep in mind that just because a product claims to be natural or green doesn't mean it's perfectly safe.

Avoid products that release volatile organic compounds (VOC). VOCs can irritate the lungs, and they may increase your risk of headaches, respiratory problems, and allergic reactions. Products that may have VOCs include:

- aerosol-spray cleaning products
- air fresheners
- bleach (or products containing chlorine bleach)
- dishwashing liquids
- furniture polish
- laundry detergents
- oven cleaners
- rug and upholstery cleaners

Look for products that do not contain VOCs, fragrances, flammable ingredients, and other irritants. If you're not sure what a product's label means or if its ingredients are safe, do more research. The US EPA, or Environmental Protection Agency, maintains a list of products that meet its safer choice requirements. Use the old-fashioned methods of warm water and soap or baking soda for tougher jobs. Instead of glass cleaners, use vinegar and water to clean windows.

The Top Ten Chemicals to Avoid
Reading product labels will help you avoid dangerous chemicals before you buy them. OneGreenPlanet.org lists these ten as the ones you should always avoid, why they're so harmful, products that are likely to include them, and what to look for on product labels.

1. 1,4-Dioxane

This chemical is used to stabilize and dissolve other substances. It is found in antifreeze, cosmetics, deodorants, and shampoos. It irritates the skin, and it can increase your risk of kidney and liver damage. Besides the chemical's name, look for dioxane, diethylene dioxide, diethylene ether, glycol ethylene ether, p-dioxane, and diethylene oxide on product labels.

2. Parabens

We have already touched on parabens, but they are found in 75 to 95 percent of cosmetics. In addition to passing through the skin and entering the body without breaking down, they can mimic estrogen, which can interfere with hormone function. Look for methyl-paraben, butylparaben, ethylparaben, and isobutyl-paraben on labels.

3. Diethanolamine (DEA)

DEA compounds reduce the acidity of ingredients and create suds. They are found in cleansers, scrubs, shampoos, and soaps. They can irritate your nasal passages. Chronic exposure affects the central nervous system, kidneys, blood, and liver, which you know is responsible for removing toxins from your body. They're poisonous to marine life. Avoid products that have cocamide DEA, Lauramide DEA, and two related chemicals, MEA and TEA.

4. Triclosan

This man-made antibacterial is found in cleansers, toothpaste, and household cleaners. It irritates the skin and eyes. It may cause cancer, alter DNA, affect fertility, and produce birth defects. It is toxic to aquatic animals.

5. Phthalates

These are used as fragrances and in plastic products. They disrupt the endocrine system, and they can cause tumors, birth defects, and a reduced sperm count in males. They're also toxic to aquatic life. They're found in air fresheners, dish soap, toilet paper, medical equipment, children's toys, and more.

6. Sulfates

They are used as foaming agents and are usually produced from petroleum. They can cause skin irritation, eye damage, labored breathing, and even depression. They can damage the immune system. Synonyms for sulfates include sodium lauryl sulfate and sodium laureth sulfate. They're found in detergents, floor cleaners, engine degreasers, hair products, and toothpaste.

7. *Formaldehyde-Releasing Chemicals*

You may not find "formaldehyde" on a product label, but other chemicals release it. It can irritate the lungs, skin, and eyes. Formaldehyde kills bacteria (that's why its antimicrobial properties make it useful as a preservative), but it is also a known carcinogen. Look for words like DMDM hydantoin, diazolidinyl urea, imidazolidinyl urea, and methenamine on the labels of hair products, moisturizers, and other personal-care products.

8. *Petroleum and Mineral Oils*

Mineral oils may sound healthy, but these hydrocarbons, which come from petroleum, clog your pores and keep your skin from breathing. These chemicals are found in engine oils, pesticides, moisturizers, lotions, and other personal care products. They're even in baby oils. These chemicals are known carcinogens and are linked with breast and skin cancer. They also disrupt the endocrine system.

9. *BHA (Butylated Hydroxyanisole) and BHT (Butylated Hydroxytoluene)*

These chemicals are used to preserve and stabilize other ingredients. They may be endocrine disruptors and carcinogens. We know that they cause cancer in fish and other wildlife. They pop up in moisturizers, cosmetics, processed food, dog food, and toys.

10. *Oxybenzone*

This is a chemical additive in sunscreen, which is a UV light absorber and filter that prevents vitamin D from being absorbed by the skin. Oxybenzone may interfere with the normal function of the immune system and the endocrine system. Ironically, it may increase your risk of developing melanoma.

Less Exposure to Toxins - Less Inflammation

There are a number of ways that you can limit your body's exposure to chemicals and other toxins that cause inflammation. These are just some of the options to reduce or eliminate the toxic heavy hitters in your environment.

For more information on ways to reduce your exposure to toxins and make the world a healthier place, check out the EPA's website. These kinds of changes often have little impact on your comfort and lifestyle, but they will have a great impact on you personally. Then, you'll be on the way to a healthier overall body.

Chapter 6
Choose the Right Foods and Drink

Step Two of the Extinguish the Flame Program

Let food be thy medicine, and medicine be thy food.

- Hippocrates

In the last chapter, you learned about the first step of the *Extinguish the Flame Program*: avoiding toxins whenever reasonably possible. This second step, choosing the right foods and drinks, maybe what comes to mind when you are fighting inflammation. Researchers know that certain foods and drinks are pro-inflammatory while others have anti-inflammatory properties.

There's another factor to consider when it comes to your diet. What and how much you eat are prime determinants of whether or not you have belly fat. Yes, the amount of exercise you do, the amount of muscle you have (which helps determine your metabolic rate or the number of calories you need to survive, even at rest), and whether your lifestyle is active or sedentary have impacts on your overall amount of body fat.

But genetics aside (you likely have a body shape that's similar to one of your parents), the foods and drinks will make the biggest difference in whether you're a healthy weight or not, and more importantly, whether you have too much fat stored around your abdomen.

Changing your diet to combat inflammation includes four basic strategies:

1. avoid foods that trigger inflammation
2. consume more foods that fight inflammation
3. manage your overall caloric intake by watching your portions
4. maintain adequate hydration

Let's look at each of these four strategies.

Say No! Avoid Common Inflammatory Foods

What's the bad news? You're probably consuming many foods that are pro-inflammatory as part of your regular diet. Fortunately, once you've identified these foods, you can work on eliminating or at least reducing your consumption of them.

Some foods are pro-inflammatory across the board, while others may trigger inflammation in some people and not in others. You may want to err on the side of caution. Take gluten. I've found that many people aren't aware that they're sensitive to it, yet when they eliminate it from their diets, their aches and pains disappear, and they feel better. If you're not sure whether a particular food is the culprit, try an elimination diet and see how you feel (See the section titled, "The Elimination Diet: Determining Your Food Sensitivities" on page 86).

Here are twelve pro-inflammatory foods and beverages to avoid:

- *Dairy Foods*

Dairy foods tend to be inflammatory. Many people can't digest the lactose and the casein that these foods contain. Most milk in the US comes from lactating cows, which are often given hormones and antibiotics. These are passed along in the milk you drink. They can impact your hormone levels and disrupt the delicate balance of healthy bacteria in the gut, leading to leaky gut syndrome. Avoid these foods, especially if you have arthritis or other joint problems.

There are some exceptions to dairy. Organic grass-fed A2/A2 milk, butter, yogurt, kefir, and cheese, and more recently, A2/A2 whey protein powders. Originally, cow's milk only had the A2 beta-casein protein present (A2/A2). This is the same primary protein found in mothers' milk, which makes it the most readily absorbed by the human body. Over time, the protein in cow's milk changed due to a genetic mutation in the A2 beta-casein. This resulted in an A1 beta-casein variant. The majority of milk in the market today is A2/A1 beta-casein, which makes it difficult to digest and can lead to inflammation and a myriad of digestive disorders or other health-related issues.

- *Soy Products*

Soy products are gaining popularity, especially among vegetarians and vegans, but they promote inflammation. The phytic acid in soy can impair nutrient absorption and irritate the lining of the gut. Soy's goitrogenic and estrogenic properties may promote thyroid and breast cancer as well.

- *Nightshades*

Many people are sensitive to the Solanaceae class of vegetables, which includes eggplants, peppers, potatoes, and tomatoes. They can cause joint pain, muscle aches, and mood swings. In addition, they promote inflammation. Limit or eliminate these if you are experiencing inflammation.

- *Gluten-Containing Foods*

These are a major contributing factor to inflammation. They include foods that contain wheat, barley, rye, and many other grains. While only a small portion of the population has celiac disease, tens of millions more are sensitive to the proteins found in the grains, which contribute to infla-mmation and leaky gut. I suggest that you avoid gluten whenever you can or at least try eliminating it from your diet before adding it back to see how you feel. As your gut heals and inflammation decreases, you may try adding one at a time back into your diet, but make sure they are organic, non-GMO, and without pesticides and chemicals whose names you cannot pronounce.

- *Alcohol*

While there is some research to suggest that a moderate amount of red wine (a glass a day) may have some cardio-vascular-protective effects, alcohol is known to trigger inflammation. It also taxes the liver, and it can throw the microbiome off balance, increasing bacterial overgrowth, which then leads to a leaky gut. It's best to consume alcohol in moderation or avoid it altogether, especially if you are experiencing unexplained inflammation.

- *Meat*

A diet high in meat is pro-inflammatory, particularly if those meats are processed or full of nitrates and other fillers. Consuming processed meat and/or eating too much fatty red meat results in high levels of arachidonic acid, which suppresses the immune system. If you are going to consume beef, make sure it is organic grass-fed. Organic chicken, turkey, and wild-caught fish are also excellent sources of protein. More about that in this chapter.

- *Sugar*

As you saw in Chapter 2, sugar is a huge player in increasing inflammation. It's a source of extra unnecessary calories, which promotes obesity and diabetes. It also compromises immune function and promotes a leaky gut.

- *Processed Foods*

Processed foods make up a whopping 50 percent of the typical American's diet. The white flour, white rice, and sugar (there's sugar again!) in these foods promote inflammation. Avoid them whenever you can.

- *Most Vegetable Oils*

Vegetable oils containing omega-6 fatty acids (such as canola, corn, and soy) cause inflammation. They also throw the ratio of omega-6 to omega-3 fatty acids out of whack. A ratio of about three omega-6 fatty acids to one omega-3 fatty acid is considered healthy, but the SAD ratio is closer to twenty to one or even higher. Avoiding fried foods whenever possible is a simple way to cut many of these oils out of your diet.

- *Caffeine-Containing Foods*

Caffeine is ubiquitous today. It shows up in everything: coffee, water, and soda. Too much of it increases your levels of stress hormones and insulin, and promotes inflammation.

- *Genetically Modified Foods*

In the modern American diet, many foods undergo genetic modification, a process that can impact their nutritional composition and, in some cases, contribute to inflammation. Genetically modified organisms (GMOs) are often designed to resist pests or enhance growth, but their long-term effects on human health are still a subject of ongoing research. Moreover, GMOs are frequently associated with the use of pesticides like glyphosate. The combination of genetically modified foods and pesticide exposure may escalate inflammation in the gastrointestinal tract, potentially leading to leaky gut syndrome.

- *Lectin-Containing Foods*

Foods like nightshades, legumes (beans, lentils, peas, and peanuts), grains, corn, and grains all contain lectins, which are proteins that may contribute to inflammation if you're sensitive to them.

> ### *The Plant Paradox: Should You Avoid Lectins?*
> You may have heard of *The Plant Paradox*. That's the title of a bestselling book published by Dr. Steven Gundry in 2017. His claim is that lectin-containing foods cause inflammation and that inflammation, in turn, causes weight gain and even obesity. If you follow his diet plan, which eliminates all lectin-containing foods, you'll have a healthier gut and lose excess body fat in the process.
>
> While people who follow Gundry's plan lose weight, it's unclear whether that's because they're avoiding lectins or because they're simply consuming fewer starchy foods, sugar, refined carbohydrates, unhealthy fats, alcohol, GMO foods, glyphosate, caffeine, and taking in fewer calories overall, resulting in weight loss. What is the bottom line? Lectins may trigger inflammation in some people. If you think that you may be sensitive to them, try an elimination diet and see how you feel when you avoid them.

FODMAP Diet

The FODMAP diet has gained recognition as a valuable approach for individuals grappling with digestive issues. FODMAPs, which stand for Fermentable Oligo-saccharides, Disaccharides, Monosaccharides, and Polyols, are specific types of carbohydrates that can trigger digestive discomfort in some people. By understanding and selectively restricting high-FODMAP foods, individuals can often manage symptoms related to conditions such as irritable bowel syndrome (IBS). Exploring the principles of the FODMAP diet may offer insights into improving digestive well-being and minimizing inflammation associated with certain carbohydrate intolerances.

Mediterranean Diet

The Mediterranean diet is known for its emphasis on fresh, whole foods and healthy fats. Rooted in the traditional eating patterns of countries bordering the Mediterranean Sea, it offers a holistic and heart-healthy approach to nourishment. Focused on fresh, whole foods rich in fruits, vegetables, olive oil, and lean proteins, this dietary lifestyle emphasizes not only flavor but also a myriad of health benefits. Explore the principles of the Mediterranean Diet to discover a balanced and sustainable way of eating, associated with reduced inflammation, improved cardiovascular health, and overall well-being.

Here are some detailed examples of meals inspired by the Mediterranean diet:

- Mediterranean Salad:

Ingredients:
- mixed greens (spinach, arugula, kale)
- cherry tomatoes
- cucumbers
- red onions
- kalamata olives
- feta cheese
- extra virgin olive oil and balsamic vinegar for dressing

- Grilled Mediterranean Chicken:

Ingredients:
- skinless, boneless chicken breast
- lemon juice
- garlic (minced)
- fresh oregano and rosemary
- olive oil
- salt and pepper

Instructions:

Marinate chicken in a mixture of lemon juice, minced garlic, chopped herbs, olive oil, salt, and pepper. Grill until fully cooked.

- Mediterranean Quinoa Bowl:

Ingredients:

- cooked quinoa
- cherry tomatoes
- cucumbers
- red bell peppers
- chickpeas (canned, rinsed)

Here are detailed recipes for two Mediterranean-inspired dishes:

- Mediterranean Chickpea Salad:

Ingredients:

- 1 can (15 oz) chickpeas, drained and rinsed
- 1 cup cherry tomatoes, halved
- 1 cucumber, diced
- 1/2 red onion, finely chopped
- 1/2 cup Kalamata olives, pitted and sliced
- 1/2 cup feta cheese, crumbled
- 1/4 cup fresh parsley, chopped

For the Dressing:

- 3 tablespoons extra virgin olive oil
- 2 tablespoons red wine vinegar, apple cider vinegar, or fresh squeezed lemon juice
- 1 clove garlic, minced
- 1 teaspoon dried oregano
- Salt and pepper to taste

Instructions:

1. In a large bowl, combine chickpeas, cherry tomatoes, cucumber, red onion, olives, feta cheese, and parsley.
2. In a small bowl, whisk together the olive oil, red wine vinegar, minced garlic, dried oregano, salt, and pepper.
3. Pour the dressing over the salad and toss gently to combine.
4. Refrigerate for at least 30 minutes before serving to let the flavors meld.

- Grilled Mediterranean Lemon Herb Chicken:

Ingredients:

  o 4 boneless, skinless chicken breasts
  o juice of 2 lemons
  o 3 cloves garlic, minced
  o 2 teaspoons dried oregano
  o 1 teaspoon dried thyme
  o 1/4 cup extra virgin olive oil
  o salt and pepper, to taste

Instructions:

1. In a bowl, mix together lemon juice, minced garlic, dried oregano, dried thyme, olive oil, salt, and pepper to create the marinade.
2. Place chicken breasts in a Ziploc bag and pour the marinade over them. Seal the bag and massage to coat the chicken. Marinate in the refrigerator for at least one hour.
3. Preheat the grill to medium high heat.
4. Grill the chicken breasts for about 6-8 minutes per side or until fully cooked.
5. Serve the grilled chicken with a side of Mediterranean chickpea salad for a complete meal.

These recipes incorporate fresh ingredients and the characteristic flavors of the Mediterranean diet. Adjust quantities to suit your preferences, and enjoy these nutritious and delicious dishes!

The Elimination Diet: Determining Your Food Sensitivities

When I treated patients with a variety of health complaints, I often suggested that they try an elimination diet to determine whether certain foods were the culprit. Everyone's biochemistry is different, and food sensitivities can cause a variety of symptoms, not all of which are digestive-related. Headaches, skin rashes, joint pain, and other symptoms may all be the result of what's on your plate.

Today, most foods consumed in America are genetically-modified and contain a number of pesticides, including glyphosate, which contribute to inflammation of the gastrointestinal tract and can lead to leaky gut syndrome. Leaky gut syndrome occurs when the integrity of the gut lining is compromised, allowing substances to leak into the bloodstream that would normally be filtered out. This condition is associated with various health issues, as the immune system may react to these leaked substances, potentially contributing to systemic inflammation and other health concerns.

Chronic gastrointestinal distress is often a symptom of some type of food intolerance. If you suspect a certain food (or more than one) is causing a problem, cut it from your diet for two weeks to see how you feel. Some of the most common culprits include dairy products, gluten-containing foods, soy, nuts, peanuts, and sugar. Not surprisingly, all of these can be pro-inflammatory. You may also want to try eliminating alcohol, caffeine, or artificial sweeteners. Make sure that you avoid the food for a full two weeks.

The easiest way to avoid any possible trigger foods is to base your diet on whole, preferably organic, non-processed foods like:

- brown rice
- chicken, turkey, and lamb
- cold-pressed coconut, avocado, or olive oil
- omega-3-containing fatty fish (albacore tuna, halibut, lake trout, mackerel, salmon, and sardines)
- fresh berries
- lightly steamed vegetables

After two weeks, you can test foods to see how they make you feel. Add one back into your diet every three days, paying attention to any symptoms you have. It may take up to three days to react to a food. This will help you identify any foods that you have difficulty digesting and avoid them in the future.

How Much Sweet Poison Do You Consume? The Leading Sources of Sugar

As you saw in Chapter 2, we eat too much sugar. Much of it is in processed foods. According to the United States Department of Agriculture, about 15 percent of daily calories come from added sugars. That's the equivalent of twenty-two teaspoons of added sugars every day! The leading sources of added sugars are:

- cakes
- candy
- cookies
- donuts and pastries
- energy and sports drinks
- fruit drinks
- ice cream and other dairy-based desserts
- pies and cobblers
- soft drinks

A food can be high in added sugar without the word *sugar* appearing on its label. Look for these names of added sugars:

- anhydrous dextrose
- brown sugar
- confectioner's powdered sugar
- corn syrup
- corn syrup solids
- dextrose
- fructose
- high-fructose corn syrup
- honey
- invert sugar
- lactose
- malt syrup
- maltose
- maple syrup
- molasses
- nectars (peach and pear)
- pancake syrup
- raw sugar
- sucrose

The easiest way to cut sugar from your diet is to eliminate soft drinks and other sweetened beverages. Replacing those drinks with water (more about that later in this chapter) will help you stay hydrated without all of the extra sugar and calories. Limiting desserts, ice cream, refined carbohydrates, and other sweets will also help you cut out the sweet poison.

Say Yes to More Plants and Less Meat: The Best Diet to Fight Inflammation

Knowing what foods to avoid or cut back on will help you combat inflammation. But you can go further by choosing foods that actually fight it.

When it comes to diet, it's hard to reach a consensus on the one that is the healthiest. Whether you choose a vegan,

Paleo, low-carb, or low-fat diet, each program has its avid proponents — and detractors. Based on all of the available research at this time, it appears that the Mediterranean diet is best when it comes to fighting inflammation. It also appears to help reduce your risk of developing cardiovascular disease, type 2 diabetes, and other health problems.

In short, the Mediterranean diet has far less meat, processed foods, and simple carbohydrates (things like cookies, candy, and other sweets) than the typical SAD. It includes more plants and monounsaturated (healthy fat) than the SAD. It has less saturated fat and less trans fat overall. It's relatively easy to eat this way when you follow these five guidelines.

- *Eat More Plant-Based Foods*

Consume more vegetables, fruits, and whole grains as part of your regular diet. However, if you suffer from chronic gastrointestinal distress, you may want to avoid gluten-containing grains or lectin-containing foods. These will be your main sources of carbohydrates, which your body uses for energy. Choose meals that are based around plants (like vegetarian chili) instead of making meat the centerpiece of every meal.

- *Eat Less Meat*

You already know meat can contribute to inflammation if consumed in excess. Avoid processed meats. Choose lean, less-fatty, preferably organic grass-fed types of meat like flank steak, bison, chicken, and lean turkey. Meat is a good source of protein when consuming organic grass-fed, but you can also get protein from non-animal sources like beans, legumes, nuts, some grains, and protein powders (preferably plant-based or organic grass-fed A2/A2 whey protein).

- *Eat More Fatty Fish*

Choose fatty fish (preferably wild and not farm-raised) like halibut, mackerel, salmon, and tuna. Opt for low-level mercury tuna, as it can contain higher levels than many other fish. These types of fish are higher in omega-3 fats than other fish. Omega-3 fatty acids combat inflammation and help create a healthier omega-6 to omega-3 ratio. Fish is another excellent source of protein.

- *Eat Fewer Dairy Products*

Some versions of the Mediterranean diet eliminate all dairy foods. Others allow low-fat or fat-free varieties. I suggest avoiding dairy if you know that you're sensitive to it. As stated earlier in Chapter 6, organic grass-fed A2/A2 dairy products are well tolerated by most people, unlike traditional A2/A1 dairy products. It's wise to experiment with A2/A2 dairy products if you are introducing it into your diet for the first time.

- *Eat More Nuts*

Nuts and seeds, especially almonds, chia seeds, flax seeds, and walnuts, are rich in phytonutrients and are a good source of healthy fats, including omega-3 fatty acids. They also help lower cholesterol and inflammatory biomarkers. Whenever possible, choose organic dry-roasted nuts without added oils. However, you may have to eliminate nuts from your diet, depending on your health condition and sensitivities. Consult with your healthcare provider for further guidance.

The Power of Protein: How Much Do You Need?

You get the calories you need from three types of macronutrients: protein, carbohydrates (carbs), and fat. Protein is made from amino acids and is one of the body's main building blocks; it's found in every cell of your body.

The amount of protein you need depends on your age, gender (men typically need a little more than women do), muscle mass, weight, state of health, and level of activity. Athletes, people who exercise a lot, and people who are trying to add muscle need more protein than others do.

A good rule of thumb for healthy adults to estimate your body's protein needs is 0.8-1 gram per kilogram of body weight. So, a 150-pound (68 kg) person would aim for 55-68 grams of protein a day, and a 200-pound (91 kg) person would need 73-91 grams. A more active adult or someone looking to build muscle mass may need a higher amount of protein. This could typically range from 1.2 to 2.2 grams per kg of body weight, depending on their specific goals or activity levels. Pregnant women require more protein, ranging from 75-100 grams per day for the developing fetus. If you eat protein at every meal, you should have no trouble reaching these guidelines. It's essential to remember that protein needs can vary significantly from person to person, and factors such as age, muscle mass, metabolic rate, and overall health goals should be considered when estimating protein requirements. Consulting with a healthcare provider or registered dietitian can provide personalized guidance on determining the best method for estimating your body's protein needs.

Quality matters just as much as, if not more, than quantity. Try to avoid meats and animal products produced by factory farms, as they are full of antibiotics and synthetic hormones. Also, take a pass on processed meats like lunchmeat, most deli meats, sausages, hot dogs, and meats served at fast-food restaurants. High-quality sources of protein include:

- beans and lentils
- lean meats and poultry, preferably from free-range animals
- grass-fed beef
- fish, particularly cold-water and wild-caught salmon, tuna, mackerel, and trout (avoid tilapia unless it's wild-caught, as it is often farmed, and contains small amounts of healthy omega-3 fats compared to the wild version)

- unsweetened, nonfat Greek-style yogurt and low-fat cottage cheese (if you have no problems with dairy, A2/A2 dairy if possible)
- eggs from free-range chickens (check the labels and buy cage-free, hormone-free organic eggs)
- raw, unsalted dry roasted nuts, especially almonds, cashews, and walnuts (preferably organic)
- nut butter (check the label to make sure that nuts are the only ingredient)
- vegan proteins from peas, rice, chia, and hemp (preferably organic or organic grass-fed A2/A2 whey protein)

Fiber Is No Fad: How to Get More into Your Diet

As a nation, we lag behind on fiber consumption. The average person consumes only fifteen grams a day, and we need twenty-five to thirty-five grams a day (That's a far cry from our hunter-gatherer ancestors, who averaged seventy-five to one hundred grams a day!).

Fiber comes in two types: insoluble and soluble. Insoluble fiber helps move the food through the gut. Soluble fiber helps replenish and feed the healthy bacteria in the gut, which is the home of 70 percent of our immune system. Fiber helps your gut fight inflammation and avoids leaky gut. It also helps slow down the digestion of carbohydrates, lowering the impact that they have on blood sugar.

Good sources of fiber include:

- fruits
- vegetables
- apple and baobab fruit fiber (are high in pectin, a soluble fiber, and can be added to food)
- gluten-free grains
- chia, hemp, and flax seeds (whole and ground)
- resistant prebiotic fibers (cassava root, soluble tapioca fiber, inulin, hydrolyzed guar fiber, and

acacia fiber, which resists breakdown in the upper gastrointestinal tract and provides food to the healthy bacteria in the lower gastrointestinal tract)

Fortunately, following the guidelines of the *Extinguish the Flame Program* will help ensure that you get enough fiber for optimal digestion and a healthier gut.

Manage Your Portions: Eating the Right Amounts of the Right Foods

Now that you know the foods to eat more of and to avoid, you're all set, right? Well, you're close. Following the *Extinguish the Flame Program's* guidelines will set you on the right path nutrition-wise, but you'll also want to make sure you're taking in the appropriate number of calories. Don't worry. You won't have to measure your food with cups or spoons. Eyeballing your portions can help you stay on track without having to count every calorie.

That can be challenging, as portions have grown over the last couple of decades. One gluten-free bagel may be the equivalent of three or four portions of bread. A restaurant entrée is often three times (or more) larger than what a typical portion should include.

It's easy to overeat even healthy foods if you're not paying attention to the size of your portions. To keep them in check, try the following:

- *Opt for Smaller Plates and Bowls*

Choosing smaller-scale dishes can lead to eating less while still feeling satisfied. Consider swapping out larger dinner plates for smaller ones to naturally control portion sizes without conscious effort.

- *Share or Save*

When dining out, consider splitting an entrée with a friend or requesting only half to be served, with the remainder wrapped for later consumption.

- *Portion Control with Prepackaging*

For foods bought in bulk, such as raw unsalted almonds, pre-measure single servings and store them in glass containers for convenient, calorie-controlled snacks.

- *Mindful Eating*

Avoid distractions like checking your phone or watching TV while eating. Taking time to focus on and savor your food can lead to consuming less and enjoying meals more.

In terms of meal composition, the Mediterranean diet provides flexibility. To promote weight loss and adhere to healthy portion sizes, consider the following meal guidelines:

- o include one serving (approximately three to four ounces) of lean protein
- o add one serving (about 1/2 cup) of high-fiber carbohydrates and/or low-glycemic-index fruits
- o incorporate one serving of healthy fats (e.g., 1 teaspoon of olive oil, 1 tablespoon of almond butter, or 1/4 cup of walnuts)
- o include one or two servings (1 to 2 cups) or more of non-starchy vegetables and leafy greens; these low-calorie, high-fiber foods help fill you up without excess calories

Here are examples of meals that meet the guidelines of Extinguish the Flame Program:

Breakfast
- o organic pasture-fed eggs, avocado, fresh berries,

- organic grass-fed A2/A2 yogurt with organic fresh berries and organic chia, flax, or hemp seeds

In a hurry and on the go, a delicious smoothie may be another option. Get creative; here is a suggestion.

Prepare a smoothie with organic plant-based protein or A2/A2 organic whey protein, organic blueberries, raspberries, strawberries, blackberries, organic almond butter, flax seeds, hemp or chia seeds, gluten-free oats, acacia fiber or hydrolyzed guar fiber, and organic coconut, oat, or almond milk.

This smoothie is nutrient-dense and rich in protein, vitamins, and antioxidants. It's a great way to kick-start your day with a healthy and satisfying breakfast. Adjust the ingredients based on your taste preferences and nutritional needs.

Lunch
Prepare a salad with organic mixed greens (arugula and red butter leaf are my favorites), cucumbers, celery, carrots, tomatoes, bell peppers, mushrooms, organic chicken breast, sunflower seeds, strawberries, and organic extra virgin cold-pressed olive oil, with lemon juice or apple cider vinegar.

Dinner
Enjoy wild-caught salmon with quinoa, broccoli, cauliflower, and carrots mixed together and drizzled with coconut oil.

Another one of my favorites is to steam organic broccoli, cauliflower, carrots, zucchini, and mushrooms. Scramble organic grass-fed eggs or organic chicken and sauté together with veggies while adding equal parts of organic extra virgin cold-pressed olive oil and organic balsamic vinegar.

Remember, nobody is perfect. Following the Mediterranean diet and avoiding inflammatory foods doesn't mean complete abstinence from occasional indulgences. Consider incurporating a cheat meal into your routine, perhaps once a week, to prevent feelings of deprivation. Moderation is key, and making gradual, sustainable changes to your diet is more effective than attempting perfection. Reward yourself occasionally with your favorite treats, fostering a balance between indulgence and maintaining a healthy lifestyle.

The concept of moderation is what you want to embrace. Think about what aspects of your diet you can change and be reasonable. It's very difficult to completely overhaul your diet and be able to stick with it. You're better off, in the long run, making small changes (swapping chips for a piece of fruit with your lunch or adding more vegetables to your dinner plate every night than trying to be perfect all of the time). If you do need to lose weight, slow but steady loss is the correct way.

I realize that not everyone has the budget for organic food, which I have included in several of the recipes. Do the best you can with your budget.

Eyeballing Portion Sizes With Your Hands

Using your hand as a reference for portion sizes is a convenient and practical way to estimate the amount of food you're consuming. Here's a general guide to measuring portion sizes with your hand:

Palm of Your Hand (Protein):
- *Men:* Typically, one palm-sized portion is equivalent to about 3-4 ounces of cooked meat, poultry, or fish.
- *Women:* A palm-sized portion is generally around 2-3 ounces.

Fist (Vegetables):
- A fist-sized portion can be used to estimate the amount of vegetables. This is a good guideline for cooked or raw vegetables.

> *Cupped Hand (Carbohydrates):*
> - A cupped hand can be used for measuring carbohydrates like rice, pasta, or other grains. A serving for women might be about one cup, while for men, it might be closer to two cups.
>
> *Thumb (Fats):*
> - The size of your thumb can be used as a reference for measuring fats and oils. This includes sources like butter, oils, or nuts. About one thumb-sized portion is a good starting point.
>
> *Finger (Snacks):*
> - When it comes to snacks, your finger can be handy. For example, one finger-sized portion of cheese or nut butter can serve as a quick snack.

It's important to note that these are rough estimates, and individual needs can vary based on factors such as age, activity level, and health goals. Additionally, the types of foods you choose can influence the overall nutritional value of your meals.

This method provides a simple way to gauge portion sizes without the need for measuring cups or scales. Keep in mind that these estimates are meant to be flexible, and adjusting based on your hunger, fullness, and specific dietary needs is encouraged. If you have specific dietary concerns or goals, consider consulting with a qualified nutrition oriented health practitioner or registered dietitian for personalized guidance.

Extinguish the Flame Program's Food
- *Non-Starchy Vegetables*

When it comes to these non-starchy vegetables, 1 cup = 1 serving. However, it is virtually impossible to consume an unhealthy amount of these veggies without feeling extremely full and unable to take another bite. Therefore, you can consume unlimited amounts of the following vegetables without going above your calorie requirement for the day.

Here's a list of non-starchy vegetables: (Remember to avoid nightshades if you think they are contributing to your inflammation.

- spinach
- kale
- broccoli
- cauliflower
- brussels sprouts
- bell peppers (all colors)
- zucchini
- cabbage
- asparagus
- green beans
- celery
- cucumber
- radishes
- tomatoes (technically a fruit, but often considered a vegetable)
- snow peas
- collard greens
- bok choy
- shallots
- water chestnuts
- artichokes

These vegetables are low in carbohydrates and can be an excellent choice for those looking to manage their blood sugar levels or reduce overall carb intake. They are also rich in vitamins, minerals, and fiber, making them a healthy addition to various meals.

- *Healthy Fats*

Here's a list of healthy fats that you can include in your diet:

- Avocado: Rich in monounsaturated fats, vitamins, and minerals.
- Olive Oil: A source of monounsaturated fats and antioxidants commonly used in Mediterranean cuisine.
- Nuts (Almonds, Walnuts, Pecans): Provide healthy fats, protein, and various nutrients.
- Seeds (Chia Seeds, Flaxseeds, Pumpkin Seeds): Good sources of omega-3 fatty acids and fiber.
- Fatty Fish (Salmon, Mackerel, Sardines): High in omega-3 fatty acids, which are beneficial for heart health.
- Coconut Oil: Contains medium-chain triglycerides (MCTs) and is suitable for cooking at high temperatures.
- Flaxseed Oil: A plant-based source of omega-3 fatty acids.
- Walnut Oil: Contains polyunsaturated fats and has a rich, nutty flavor.
- Chia Oil: High in omega-3 fatty acids and suitable for adding to salads and dressings.
- Dark Chocolate (in moderation): Provides healthy fats and antioxidants and may have some health benefits.
- Fatty Acids from Grass-Fed Meat and Dairy: Grass-fed sources may contain higher levels of omega-3 fatty acids.
- Nut Butter (Almond Butter, Peanut Butter): Choose varieties with no added sugars or unhealthy additives.
- Avocado Oil: Similar to olive oil, it is suitable for cooking or as a salad dressing.
- Sesame Oil: Contains monounsaturated and poly-unsaturated fats, commonly used in Asian cuisine.

- Olives: A good source of monounsaturated fats and antioxidants.

When incorporating fats into your diet, it's essential to focus on a balance of different types of fats and consume them in moderation as part of a well-rounded, nutritious diet.

- *Legumes and Starchy Vegetables (1/2 cup = 1 serving)*

Here's a list of legumes and healthy starchy vegetables:

Legumes:
- Chickpeas (Garbanzo Beans): Rich in protein, fiber, and various vitamins and minerals.
- Lentils: High in protein, fiber, and iron.
- Black Beans: A good source of protein, fiber, and folate.
- Kidney Beans: Contain protein, fiber, and antioxidants.
- Pinto Beans: Provide protein, fiber, and various nutrients.
- Split Peas: High in protein, fiber, and vitamin B.
- Black-eyed Peas: Rich in protein, fiber, and potassium.
- Soybeans (Edamame): A complete protein source that is rich in fiber.
- Lima Beans: Contain protein, fiber, and important minerals.
- Cannellini Beans: Provide protein, fiber, and iron.

Healthy Starchy Vegetables:
- Sweet Potatoes: Rich in beta-carotene, fiber, and vitamins.
- Butternut Squash: Contains fiber, vitamins A and C, and potassium.
- Acorn Squash: A good source of fiber, vitamin C, and potassium.
- Peas: Provide fiber, protein, and various vitamins.

- Corn: Contains fiber, vitamins, and antioxidants.
- Potatoes (especially with skin): Provide potassium, vitamin C, and fiber.
- Pumpkin: Rich in beta-carotene, fiber, and vitamins.
- Carrots: High in beta-carotene, fiber, and vitamins.
- Beets: Contain fiber, folate, and antioxidants.
- Plantains: Provide complex carbohydrates and vitamins.

When including legumes and starchy vegetables in your diet, consider their nutritional content and their place within a balanced and diverse meal plan. These foods offer valuable nutrients, including fiber, protein, and various vitamins and minerals.

- *Grains (1/2 cup = 1 serving)*

Here's a list of gluten-free grains that can be included in a gluten-free diet:

- Quinoa: A complete protein source with a nutty flavor.
- Rice (all varieties): Including brown rice, black rice, and wild rice.
- Corn: Corn and corn-based products are naturally gluten-free. Organic and non-GMO preferably.
- Millet: A small, round grain with a mild flavor.
- Amaranth: A tiny grain high in protein and fiber.
- Buckwheat: Despite its name, buckwheat is not wheat and is gluten-free. It can be used in various forms, such as groats or flour.
- Sorghum: A versatile grain with a neutral taste and is gluten-free.
- Teff: A small grain often used in Ethiopian cuisine.
- Arrowroot: A gluten-free starch commonly used as a thickening agent.

- Oats (gluten-free): While oats themselves are gluten-free, cross-contamination can occur during process-sing. Choose certified gluten-free oats if you have gluten sensitivity.
- Coconut Flour: Ground from dried coconut, it's a gluten-free alternative for baking.
- Almond Flour: Made from ground almonds, it's commonly used in gluten-free baking.
- Chickpea Flour (Garbanzo Bean Flour): High in protein, used in various culinary applications, and gluten-free.
- Cassava (Yuca): A starchy root vegetable used to make flour and various products.

When following a gluten-free diet, it's crucial to choose products labeled as gluten-free, especially for grains like oats, to avoid cross-contamination. Additionally, always check ingredient labels to ensure that gluten-containing grains are not present in processed foods.

For baking bread, muffins, pastries, or other gluten-free recipes, there are several flours like almond, amaranth, arrowroot, coconut, gluten-free oat, quinoa, rice, sorghum, or potato,

- *Fruits (1/2 cup = 1 serving, except where indicated)* Here's a list of healthy fruits that are rich in vitamins, minerals, fiber, and antioxidants:

  - Berries: blueberries, strawberries, raspberries, blackberries, cranberries
  - Citrus Fruits: oranges, grapefruits, lemons, limes, tangerines
  - Tropical Fruits: pineapple, mango, papaya, kiwi, guava
  - Stone Fruits: apples, pears, peaches, plums, cherries
  - Melons: watermelon, cantaloupe, honeydew

- Bananas: Rich in potassium and a convenient, portable snack.
- Grapes: Both red and green grapes offer antioxidants.
- Avocado: While technically a berry, avocados are often treated as a savory fruit. They are rich in healthy fats.
- Pomegranate: Known for its antioxidant properties.
- Tomatoes: Botanically a fruit, tomatoes are a good source of vitamins and antioxidants.
- Kiwi: High in vitamin C and fiber.
- Apricots: Provide vitamins A and C, as well as fiber.
- Cantaloupe: Hydrating and rich in vitamins A and C.
- Stoneless Fruits:
- Olives: High in antioxidants
- Coconut (fresh or unsweetened): High in fiber and medium-chain fatty acids, which make it easier to digest.
- Dragon Fruit (Pitaya): A tropical fruit with a vibrant appearance that is rich in antioxidants.

Remember to consume a variety of fruits to ensure a diverse range of nutrients (preferably organic without the pesticides often found on a variety of fruits). Additionally, moderation is key, as fruits contain natural sugars. If you have specific dietary considerations or health conditions, it's advisable to consult with a nutrition-oriented healthcare provider or a registered dietitian.

High glycemic fruits contain sugars that are quickly absorbed into the bloodstream, causing a rapid increase in blood sugar levels. Some examples are bananas, grapes, mangoes, papayas, pineapples, dates, and watermelon.

- *Animal Proteins (3 to 4 ounces = 1 serving)*

Here's a list of healthy animal proteins that are rich in essential nutrients like protein, vitamins, and minerals:

- Chicken Breast: Lean and versatile, a good source of protein.
- Turkey: Lean turkey, especially turkey breast, is a low-fat protein option.
- Lean Beef (Organic Grass-Fed): Provides protein, iron, and zinc.
- Eggs: A complete protein source with essential vitamins and minerals.
- Yogurt: High in protein, good source of probiotics and calcium (look for A2/A2 organic grass-fed yogurt).
- Cottage Cheese: A protein-rich dairy option that also contains calcium (look for A2/A2 organic grass-fed).
- Lean Pork (Tenderloin): Provides protein, vitamins, and minerals.
- Chicken Thighs (Skinless): Dark meat is still a good source of protein.
- Venison: Lean game meat, rich in protein and low in fat.
- Lamb (Lean Cuts): A source of protein, iron, and vitamin B12.
- Shrimp: Low in calories and high in protein.
- Crab: A lean seafood option providing protein and nutrients.
- Scallops: A low-fat shellfish option rich in protein.
- Bison: A lean alternative to beef, providing protein and iron.

- Fish and Seafood: A rich source of high-quality animal protein, omega-3 fatty acids, and various essential nutrients.

When selecting animal proteins, opt for lean cuts and incorporate a variety to ensure a diverse nutrient intake. It's also important to consider your individual dietary needs, preferences, and health conditions. Always practice proper cooking methods and food safety guidelines when preparing animal proteins.

Seafood is a rich source of high-quality protein, omega-3 fatty acids, and various essential nutrients. Here's a list of healthy seafood proteins:

- Salmon: Rich in omega-3 fatty acids, protein, and vitamin D.
- Tuna: A good source of lean protein and omega-3s.
- Mackerel: High in omega-3 fatty acids and vitamin D.
- Sardines: Packed with omega-3s, calcium, and vitamin D.
- Trout: A freshwater fish with omega-3s and protein.
- Halibut: A lean fish high in protein and various nutrients.
- Cod: Low in fat and a good source of protein.
- Shrimp: Low in calories, high in protein, and a good source of selenium.
- Crab: A low-fat seafood option with protein and nutrients.
- Scallops: Low in fat, high in protein, and a good source of magnesium.
- Oysters: Provide protein, zinc, and other essential minerals.

- Clams: A nutrient-dense seafood option with protein and iron.
- Anchovies: High in omega-3s and a good source of calcium.
- Haddock: A lean white fish with protein and various vitamins.
- Crayfish: Low in fat and calories, rich in protein.

When incorporating seafood into your diet, it's important to choose a variety of options to benefit from a diverse range of nutrients. Additionally, be mindful of sustainability and choose seafood that is responsibly sourced to support healthy marine ecosystems.

Here are some meal plans you can follow in order to maintain a healthy lifestyle:

Vegetarian Quinoa Salad:
Ingredients:

- quinoa
- cherry tomatoes
- cucumber
- bell peppers
- feta cheese (optional)
- olive oil
- lemon juice
- salt
- pepper

Lectin-Free Eggplant Lasagna:
Ingredients:

- eggplant slices
- tomato sauce (lectin-free)
- spinach
- garlic
- olive oil
- nutritional yeast

Organic Chicken Stir-Fry:
Ingredients:

- organic chicken breast
- broccoli
- bell peppers
- carrots
- gluten-free tamari sauce
- sesame oil
- ginger

Wild Caught Salmon with Lemon-Dill Sauce:
Ingredients:

- wild-caught salmon fillet
- lemon, fresh dill
- olive oil
- salt
- pepper

Dairy and Soy-Free Coconut Curry Tofu:
Ingredients:

- firm tofu
- coconut milk
- curry paste
- vegetables (e.g., bell peppers, peas, carrots)
- basmati rice

Nightshade-Free Turkey and Sweet Potato Hash:
Ingredients:

- ground turkey
- sweet potatoes
- spinach, garlic
- olive oil
- salt
- pepper

Instructions:

1. Heat olive oil in a skillet over medium heat.
2. Add ground turkey and cook until browned.
3. Add diced sweet potatoes and cook until tender.
4. Stir in chopped spinach and minced garlic, cooking until spinach wilts.
5. Season with salt and pepper to taste.
6. Serve warm.

This recipe avoids nightshade ingredients.

Vegetarian Quinoa Salad:
Ingredients:

- 1 cup quinoa
- 1 cup cherry tomatoes, halved
- 1 cucumber, diced
- 1 bell pepper, diced
- 2 tablespoons olive oil
- juice of one lemon
- salt and pepper to taste
- optional: feta cheese (lactose-free if needed)

Lectin-Free Eggplant Lasagna:
Ingredients:

- 1 large eggplant, thinly sliced
- lectin-free tomato sauce
- 2 cups fresh spinach
- 2 cloves garlic, minced
- 2 tablespoons olive oil
- nutritional yeast for topping

Organic Chicken Stir-Fry:
Ingredients:

- 1 lb. organic chicken breast, sliced
- 1 cup broccoli florets

- 1 bell pepper, sliced
- 1 cup sliced carrots
- 3 tablespoons gluten-free tamari sauce
- 2 tablespoons sesame oil
- 1 tablespoon grated ginger

Wild Caught Salmon with Lemon-Dill Sauce:
Ingredients:

- 2 wild-caught salmon fillets
- juice of one lemon
- 2 tablespoons fresh dill, chopped
- 2 tablespoons olive oil
- salt and pepper to taste

FODMAP-Friendly Quinoa Bowl:
Ingredients:

- 1 cup quinoa
- 1 zucchini, sliced
- 1 cup cherry tomatoes, halved
- 1 cup spinach
- 2 tablespoons olive oil
- juice of one lemon
- 1/4 cup pine nuts

Dairy-Free Coconut Curry Tofu:
Ingredients:

- 1 block of firm tofu, cubed
- 1 can of coconut milk
- 3 tablespoons curry paste
- mixed vegetables (bell peppers, peas, carrots)
- basmati rice for serving

Feel free to customize these recipes.

Achieve Optimal Hydration: Water is the Fountain of Youth

So far in this chapter, we've focused on food, but the final component of eating to combat inflammation isn't only about what you eat but about what you drink. Let's take a closer look at why it's so critical and how to make sure that you're properly hydrated.

You can go a few days or even longer without food. This is not true of water. Without water, everything dies. Not only does every organism need water, but every single cell needs to be properly hydrated in order to function within that organism. Each tiny, microscopic cell is full of life-giving water. When you consider that your body has trillions of cells and that about 60 percent of the human adult body is made of water, that's a lot of watering to do. Yet, as a nation, we are typically under-hydrated at best.

How much water should you consume daily? The standard rule is to take your body weight and divide it in half to determine the *minimum* number of ounces per day that you need. Therefore, a one-hundred-pound person should have a minimum of fifty ounces of water per day, just for minimal healthy function. A 125-pound person should have sixty-three ounces, a 150-pound person should have seventy-five ounces, and a two-hundred-pound person should have a minimum of one hundred ounces per day.

Consider water to be your fountain of youth. Water is first shuttled to organs to help them function and then to muscles, which, when hydrated, improve strength and flexibility. Water makes its way to the skin (the body's outer layer) only after everything else is properly hydrated. What if your body isn't so lucky? Then, you're likely to develop wrinkles and show signs of aging much earlier, inside and outside. Water helps provide that extra pep in your step and is one of the best ways to give yourself a natural facelift.

The Myth of Eight Glasses per Day

Have you heard you should drink eight glasses of water a day? There's no scientific evidence for this. The slogan and health myth of six glasses per day was first introduced to the American public in 1945. Today, eight glasses a day translates to eight 8-ounce glasses or 64 ounces total. This amount is fine if you weigh 128 pounds and aren't particularly active. You do get some fluids from foods, especially fruits and vegetables. However, as a nation, we're not eating enough of those, so this recommended amount is less than what you need.

Instead, use the half-your-body-weight standard as your minimum water intake. Monitor your urine to keep tabs on your hydration. It should be clear or light yellow. Dark or scanty urine is an indicator of under-hydration. You'll find ideas on how to track your water intake later in this chapter.

The minimum amount is for the following basic cellular and bodily functions:

- providing saliva in your mouth
- aiding digestion
- lubricating cartilage and joints
- keeping nasal passages and other mucosal membranes (like intestines) moist
- regulating your body's temperature
- acting as shock absorber for the brain and spinal cord
- manufacturing hormones and neurotransmitters in the brain
- delivering oxygen throughout the body
- keeping the kidneys and bladder functioning
- and yes, even providing lubrication for your sex life

But, when it comes to dealing with actual inflammation, water is the number one key element that flushes toxins and cellular waste from the trillions of cells in the body. That's why it's so important.

A number of factors can impact hydration: gender, age, weight, muscle mass (muscle cells require more water than fat cells do), electrolytes, stress levels, climate, illness, and amount of exercise. Typically, babies, men, pregnant women, and people with more muscle have a higher percentage of water in their bodies and, therefore, need more water for proper functioning. You may also need more water than average if you're middle-aged or older, are ill, or live in a dry climate such as Nevada, Arizona, New Mexico, Southern California, or Texas.

Do You Want to Drink More Water?
Keep a Water Log.

One of my female colleagues is a licensed massage therapist who studied hydrotherapy for one of her classes at the International School of Professional Bodywork in San Diego, California. Perhaps intuiting that most students, like most Americans, were under-hydrated, the instructor had students create written water logs for one of their course assignments. They tracked their water consumption over the course of seven days and then reported their own personal findings. They didn't change anything else about their diet or exercise routines.

The students had to commit to a hydration protocol in advance. They were given two options. One option was to follow the recommended divide-your-body-weight-in-half calculation to determine the number of ounces they would need to consume, which most students did. The other option was drinking 100 ounces per day (for women) or 120 ounces per day (for men), regardless of their body weight.

My colleague took on the latter option as a challenge and out of curiosity. Her personal findings surprised her. She reported that she had more energy throughout the day and that it greatly improved her concentration and mood (She was already happy, but she went so far as to report an extra-elevated excitement). It also reduced her lower back pain, which on some days became nonexistent, and it ever so slightly reduced the fine lines on her face. She found that she *wanted* to exercise more, but for the sake of the study, she opted not to. She looked and felt younger. All of this came after only seven days. Imagine what a whole month of hydrating this way could do for you!

Is Water the Answer for Your Digestive Problems?

Kevin, 57, had been experiencing problems with his digestion for several months. He felt bloated and heavy after meals, was constipated, and had constant dull headaches. He was eating a lot of raw vegetables, fruits, and processed carbs in the form of bread and pasta, but he was drinking very little fluids.

I told him to switch to cooked vegetables instead of raw (they're easier to digest), eliminate the processed carbs, and drink between 8 and 12 cups of fluids a day. I also recommended that he take a digestive formula.

After just two weeks, all of his symptoms had disappeared. He had no more bloating after meals, his bowel movements were regular, and his headaches had disappeared. At his follow-up visit six months later, Kevin was still free of any digestive problems.

- Wojciech Konior, MD

Simple Ways to Maintain Good Hydration
Drinking more water is mostly a matter of habit. Once you start drinking more, you'll find it becomes automatic. Give these twelve strategies a try to help you drink more.

- *Make a Favorite Glass Your Own*

Choose a stein, tumbler, water bottle, or whatever you like, and measure how much water it holds. I like to start my day with a large glass of water with freshly squeezed lemon. My favorite water bottle holds thirty-two ounces. I carry this with me throughout the day and try to consume at least two of these throughout the day in addition to my morning ritual of several glasses upon arising.

- *Track Your Water*

When you first start drinking more water, track the amount diligently on paper, a spreadsheet, or a health-related app (such as MyFitnessPal) so that you can get an accurate picture of your intake. We tend to fib to ourselves by often overestimating our good habits while downplaying our bad ones. Once you get into a rhythm and have your favorite glass, you can mentally track how much water you've had.

Have a glass of water as soon as you wake up and before your morning coffee and breakfast. Adding a squeeze of lemon is refreshing, and it goes down easier.

- *Play Games*

I like to call them *water sports*. Create a reward system for yourself. For example, allow yourself to check in with social media only after you've consumed a certain amount of water. Do you remember that little square of 70 percent dark chocolate you've been dreaming about? You can have it only after you've met your daily goal. I sometimes like to play the drink-fifty-ounces-by-noon game and often find myself chugging the rest of my bottle in the early afternoon. Do whatever works for you!

- *Avoid Buying Water in Plastic Bottles*

Not only is it terrible for the environment (plastic bottles end up in landfills), but plastic bottles also contain harmful chemicals. Glass bottles and stainless-steel containers are better for both you and the environment.

- *Use a Water Filtration System*

The National Drinking Water Database, published by the Environment Working Group, found 316 pollutants in drinking water in forty-five different states. This is all the more reason to use some sort of filtration system. It's less expensive than buying bottled water, and it may encourage you to drink more water.

If your budget allows, you can get really fancy and install a system that connects to the plumbing under your kitchen sink or to your faucet. A gravity-driven pitcher works well, too, and it is a less expensive option. It's really all about the filter, and activated carbon seems to be the best kind.

Do you want to know more about your city's water supply? Contact your local water utility.

- *Try a Steam Room or an Infrared Sauna*

They both help hydrate your skin and moisten your nasal passages. You'll sweat while you're in there, so be sure to drink extra water during and afterward. This helps move the water and impurities through your system and aids your body in the detoxification process. Indulging in a session in a steam room or an infrared sauna not only provides a relaxing escape but also offers numerous benefits for your overall well-being.

The steam in a traditional steam room and the infrared heat in saunas contribute to improved circulation, promoting a healthy glow and enhancing skin elasticity. I have personally owned an infrared sauna for over 6 years and found numerous benefits when utilizing it on a frequent basis. It seems to have shortened the duration and severity of fighting a cold or flu. I've also observed improvements in my sleep, skin, and a more calming effect under stressful situations.

Here's an overview of some potential health benefits of infrared saunas supported by scientific studies:

- Detoxification:
    - Some studies suggest that infrared saunas may help with detoxification by promoting sweating and the elimination of certain toxins through the skin.
- Cardiovascular Health:
    - Research indicates that regular use of infrared saunas may have positive effects on Cardiovascular health, such as improving blood pressure and enhancing blood vessel function.
- Pain Relief:
    - Infrared sauna sessions have been associated with reduced pain in conditions like arthritis and musculoskeletal disorders. The heat from the sauna may help alleviate discomfort.
- Relaxation and Stress Reduction:
    - Infrared sauna use may contribute to relaxation and stress reduction. Studies suggest a potential positive impact on cortisol levels, indicating a stress-reducing effect.
- Skin Health:
    - The heat from infrared saunas may promote improved skin health, including enhanced circulation, reduced signs of aging, and potential benefits for certain skin conditions.
- Improved Sleep:
    - Some individuals report improved sleep quality as a result of regular infrared sauna sessions. The relaxation induced by the sauna's heat may contribute to better sleep.

- Weight Loss:
    - While not a replacement for diet and exercise, some studies suggest that infrared saunas may contribute to weight loss through increased calorie expenditure and improved metabolic function.

It's important to note that while there is research supporting these potential benefits, individual responses to infrared sauna therapy may vary. Always consult with a healthcare provider, especially if you have pre-existing health conditions.

- *Take a Bath with Epsom Salt*

Enjoy a cup of warm herbal tea, which doesn't contain caffeine, as you bathe. Epsom salt can help your body absorb magnesium, which is an essential mineral, through your skin, ease sore muscles, and reduce inflammation. Make sure you hydrate afterward. An Epsom salt bath is a wonderful way to unwind and relieve stress.

- *Consider Using a Humidifier*

If you live in a dry climate, a humidifier will add more moisture to the air in your home. If this isn't within your budget, create your own by boiling water on your stove (Never leave it unattended). Add some peels from lemons, limes, or oranges, and voilà! You have your own natural aromatherapy and room deodorizer. A humidifier won't improve your body's overall hydration, but it will help soothe dry skin and nasal passages in extra-dry climates.

- *Eat More Hydrating Foods*

Fruits and vegetables contain a lot of water, along with vitamins, minerals, phytonutrients, and electrolytes. Electrolytes will help you maintain the appropriate balance of fluids in your body.

- *Infuse Your Water*

If you find plain old water boring, add some fresh fruits or herbs to it. Wash everything thoroughly. Slice or dice the fruit. Smack the herbs against the palm of your hand to bring out their essence. This breaks open the capillaries in the plants' tissues and releases their delicious herbal essence. Add these to your water, and every sip will be like a scrumptious aromatherapy session for you.

Some ideas that you might like to try would be strawberry and basil, cucumber and melon, lemon and rosemary, pineapple and kiwi, or lime and cilantro. You can also add a healthy, no-calorie sweetener like stevia or monk fruit to make your drink more desirable.

- *Front Load Your Water Consumption*

Try to drink all of your water earlier in the day. I try to get most of my water in by 6:00 p.m. That way, you don't have to get up to use the restroom in the middle of the night, which interrupts your sleep.

In short, water is essential for achieving and maintaining optimal health. I believe it's what flows in the fountain of youth. It's the source of well-being and vitality. It's a natural elixir and energizer. Getting enough will help you hydrate your way to health. That's the final aspect of eating in the *Extinguish the Flame Program*.

Circadian Rhythms

Nutrition scientists have long debated the ideal diet for achieving optimal health. Now, some experts believe it's not only what we eat that's critical for our good health but also when we eat it.

There is a growing body of evidence to suggest that our bodies function optimally when we align our eating patterns with our circadian rhythms, which is the innate twenty-four-hour cycle (our body's built-in clock) that tells us when to wake up, when to eat, and when to fall asleep.

Studies show that disrupting this rhythm by eating dinner and drinking late in the evening or grabbing a midnight snack could be a recipe for weight gain, obesity, depression, anxiety, diabetes, high blood pressure, high cholesterol, fatty liver disease, acid reflux, heart attack, cancer, Alzheimer's disease, and more

In fact, circadian rhythms control our hormones, brain chemicals, enzymes, and even the microbes found in our gut. Research has shown that eating within a ten-to-twelve-hour window during the first half of the day is best for your circadian rhythm.

For example, eat a healthy breakfast at 7:00 a.m. and your last meal at 5:00 p.m. This is the optimal time window for our bodies to digest food and absorb nutrients. Any later, our bodies will be spending an enormous amount of energy digesting food when they should be slowing down in preparation for sleep.

In addition, Dr. Satchin Panda, author of *The Circadian Code,* suggests three steps for maintaining a healthy circadian rhythm in order to give the body time to repair and rejuvenate.

1. get outside for 30 minutes every morning to get the proper amount of light
2. consume all of your food over a span of 8–12 hours, starting first thing in the morning
3. spend at least eight hours in bed sleeping, depending on your age

See Chapter 9, "Better Sleep, Better Health," for more information.

Chapter 7
Move Your Body More

Step Three of the Extinguish the Flame Program

Changing your diet so that you're eating fewer inflammatory foods and more foods that fight inflammation takes a fair number of conscious choices — at least in the beginning. As these choices become habits, you'll find it easier to maintain them without having to think about them. Keep that in mind as you learn about the third step of the *Extinguish the Flame Program*: becoming more active.

This is a hard sell for many of the people that I have treated. People say that they're too busy to exercise, they can't afford an expensive gym membership, or they simply don't like to sweat. There's no shortage of excuses when it comes to failing to exercise, but the fact is that a sedentary lifestyle promotes inflammation. Moving your body more helps combat it. You don't have to be a weekend warrior or spend hours at the gym to become more active.

Moving more includes the following three strategies:

1. Do strength-building exercises two or three times a week.
2. Get aerobic exercise three or four times a week.
3. Move more throughout the day.

That's it! Let's look at each of these strategies and ways to implement them.

The Connection between Inflammation and Inactivity

At this point, everyone knows that you're supposed to exercise and that it's good for your overall health. Physical activity helps lower bad cholesterol while raising good cholesterol. It helps prevent heart disease, type 2 diabetes, and many forms of cancer, including breast cancer. It improves the strength of your bones, muscles, and joints and your self-esteem, combats depression and anxiety, and helps you sleep better.

The activity also helps fight inflammation. When you exercise, your muscle cells release a specific protein called interleukin 6, which helps lower the levels of other proteins (TNF alpha and interleukin 1) that trigger inflammation. In other words, exercise helps you turn your inflammatory switch *off*.

We are not designed to sit around staring at screens or punching texts into smartphones. Our bodies are made to move and to move often. Researchers may not have yet determined the perfect dose of exercise in terms of reducing inflammation (and that may vary depending on your age and biochemistry), but staying active and doing exercise that builds muscle (strength training) along with exercise that puts additional demands on your cardiovascular system (aerobic exercise or cardio), all help counter inflammation.

Besides that, it feels good to move. You played games and ran around outside as a kid with no thought of health benefits. It was just fun! (I wrote more about play and its importance in Chapter 8). In an increasingly sedentary society, you can now go all day without breathing hard or challenging your body in any way, and that's a drain on your overall health, your energy, and even your mood.

It's important to note that you can have too much of a good thing. Over-exercise, such as when you train hard day after day with no chance for your body to recover, promotes inflammation. People who run ultramarathons (races that are longer than 26.2 miles) and those who can't live without a hard workout most days of the week may not be doing their bodies any favors, but they're in the minority. Most of us need to move more often and intentionally so that we can help our bodies fight off chronic inflammation.

> ### *When You Can't Exercise*
>
> Exercise helps combat inflammation, but what happens when you're too inflamed to exercise? You may have to focus on the other steps of the Extinguish the Flame Program and ease your way into becoming more active.
>
> Molly, age 44, had signs of significant inflammation, including an enlarged heart, asthma, psoriasis on both of her legs, and extreme fatigue. She had difficulty breathing and couldn't exercise as a result.
>
> She started following a gluten-free, dairy-free, and low-sugar diet and drinking more water. She also started taking supplements that included omega-3 fish oil, coenzyme Q10, turmeric, Boswellia, ginger, B complex vitamin, and glutamine. Several months later, her asthma had improved so much that she was able to exercise regularly and no longer needed to nap continuously. And her psoriasis skin condition was completely gone on one leg, and 85 percent improved on the other.
>
> - Coreen Reinhart, CCN

Make the Most of Your Muscles: Why Strength Training Matters

Exercise fads come and go. From the running boom of the seventies to the Jane Fonda era of bodysuits and legwarmers in the eighties to the CrossFit culture of today, there's always some trendy way to work out. But the bottom line is that the most effective exercise you can do doesn't require any special clothes, instruction, or equipment. You need minimal equipment, some household items like heavy canned goods, and a set or two of dumbbells to get started.

Strengthening your muscles pays off in a number of ways. First off, it boosts your metabolism, which means you burn more calories all the time. It reduces your risk of developing type 2 diabetes. It also helps you retain bone mass and reduces your risk of osteoporosis. It can help boost self-confidence and reduce your risk of injury.

It can make all of your day-to-day tasks easier, whether that's unloading heavy bags of groceries or mowing the grass. Using your muscles helps make your body more sensitive to insulin, which means you're less likely to store extra calories as fat, including belly fat, which we know is an inflammation trigger.

Muscle matters, and you want to keep yours. Both men and women typically begin to lose some muscle mass in their thirties unless they strength-train or otherwise challenge their muscles on a regular basis. That's scary, but the good news is that this loss is reversible. Even seniors in their sixties and beyond can build and retain muscle by lifting weights regularly.

The key is challenging your muscles beyond what they're used to. When you do this, you create micro-tears in the muscle, which your body then repairs over the next day or two. The result is stronger, denser muscles. If you train regularly, you may also see an increase in muscle size, which is called hypertrophy. Ladies, don't worry. You won't become muscle-bound. This is a popular but unfounded myth in regard to weightlifting.

You'll find a complete workout below, which will target all of your major muscle groups. Keep the following tips in mind for a safe, effective strength-training workout:

- Warm up by walking, biking, or doing other aerobic activities five to ten minutes before you lift weights. This will raise your heart rate, increase blood flow to your muscles, and let you mentally gear up for your workout.
- Form is more important than the amount of weight you lift. You want to do the moves in a slow, controlled fashion and without jerking or changing your body's position. If you can't do another repetition while maintaining good form, stop.
- Breathe normally as you lift weights, inhaling during the easier part of the move and exhaling during the more challenging part. For example, if you do bicep curls where you're bending your elbows to bring your knuckles to your shoulders, you'll exhale as you bring the weights up and inhale as you lower them down.
- Start with one set of eight to twelve repetitions (reps) of each exercise. At the end of the set, your muscles should feel challenged, as if it would be difficult to do another rep or two. If you feel like you could bang out another fifteen reps with no problem, either slow down (this makes it more challenging) or try a heavier weight. As you grow stronger, you can work up to two to three sets of eight to fifteen reps per exercise.
- Stabilize your core when you're doing standing exercises. In short, this means that you engage the muscles of your abdomen to help protect your back and prevent injury. Before you begin, imagine drawing your navel back toward your spine. This will engage your abs.
- Train your large muscle groups (legs, back, and chest) before your smaller muscles (biceps, triceps, and shoulders). It's also smart to train opposite muscle groups. For example, you might do a chest

press or a pushup, which involves your pushing muscles, before doing a bent-over row, which uses your back and biceps or pulling muscles.
- Focus on what you're doing. When you do cardio, it's okay to space out. However, you will get a lot more out of a strength-training session when you slow down and put your mind into your muscles.
- Have fun! Both women and men find that they enjoy strength training once they get started. A little soreness is normal at first, but that will go away as your body adjusts to the challenges you're putting on it.

The Eight-Exercise Extinguish the Flame Program Strength Routine

This routine will train all of your major muscle groups and help you get comfortable lifting weights if you haven't done it before. You'll need a heavier set of dumbbells for chest and back exercises and a lighter set for the shoulders and arms exercises. Make the moves in order.

1. Body-Weight Squat (Targets the Legs)

Stand with your feet under your hips and your toes pointed out slightly. Engage your core (Imagine drawing your navel toward your spine) and inhale as you bend your knees to push your bottom back and down (as if you were going to sit on a toilet behind you). Keep your knees behind your toes. Stop when your thighs are nearly parallel to the ground or as low as is comfortable. Exhale as you return to the starting position. That's one rep. Do eight to twelve of them. You can hold the dumbbells at your sides to make it more challenging.

2. Chest Press (Targets Chest, Shoulders, and Triceps)

Lie on your back on a bench with your feet on the floor. Your dumbbells should be in your hands at chest level, and your elbows should be bent at ninety-degree angles. Exhale as you press the dumbbells straight up toward the ceiling until your arms are straight (but without locking your elbows). Lower them back to the starting position as you inhale. That's one rep.

3. Bent-Over Row (Targets Back and Biceps)

Stand with your feet a hip distance apart while holding a dumbbell in your right hand. Bend forward at the waist so that your torso is parallel to the ground and engage your core (Imagine drawing your navel toward your spine). Exhale as you pull (or row) the dumbbell up toward your right hip, keeping it close to your body until your elbow makes a ninety-degree angle. Inhale as you lower the dumbbell back down. That's one rep.

4. Body-Weight Lunge (Targets Legs)

Stand with your feet a hip distance apart. Your arms are at your sides. Engage your core (Imagine drawing your navel toward your spine) and step your right foot forward about eighteen inches or far enough so that your right and your left knee make ninety-degree angles as you lower your right knee toward the ground. Inhale as you lower your right knee to a few inches off the ground. Keep your chest up. Then pause briefly and exhale as you step your right foot back to the starting position.

Repeat on the other side and step your left foot forward. That's one rep. You can hold dumbbells at your sides to make it more challenging.

5. Shoulder Press (Targets Shoulders)

Stand with your feet a hip distance apart and engage your core by pulling your navel toward your spine. Hold the dumbbells just above your shoulders, with your elbows bent and your knuckles facing each other. Keep your core engaged as you exhale and press the dumbbells up over your shoulders. Pause when your arms are straight, and then lower them back down to the starting position as you inhale. That's one rep.

6. Biceps Curl (Targets Biceps)

Stand with your feet a hip distance apart. Hold the dumbbells at your sides with your knuckles facing up and engage your core by pulling your navel toward your spine. Exhale as you bend your elbows to bring the dumbbells up to your shoulders while keeping your arms close to your body. Then, inhale as you lower the dumbbells back to the starting position. That's one rep.

7. Triceps Kickback (Targets Triceps)

Stand with your feet a hip distance apart while holding a dumbbell in your right hand. Bend forward at the waist so that your torso is parallel to the ground, engage your core (Imagine drawing your navel toward your spine), and bend your elbow so that it makes a ninety-degree angle. Keep your arm close to your body, and exhale as you extend your arm toward your hip until your arm is straight. Then, inhale as you return your arm to the ninety-degree angle position. That's one rep.

8. Bicycle (Targets Abdominals)

Lie on your back with your knees bent and your feet under your hips. Place your hands behind your head and interlace your fingers. Lift your feet off the ground so that your shins are parallel to the ground. Lift your head and shoulders, twist your torso slightly, and bring your right elbow toward your left knee as you extend your right leg all the way. Then, bring your left elbow toward your right knee as you extend your left leg. That's one rep. Breathe normally as you do the exercise.

Do this strength-building workout two to three times a week, increasing the weights you use as you get stronger. After six to eight weeks, you may want to mix up your routine by swapping in different exercises, which you can find in other strength-training books, or by hiring a personal trainer for a few sessions to teach you some new, more challenging moves.

Exercise Myths Debunked

Wayne, whom I speak of in this chapter, had a tendency to over-exercise, which can cause more inflammation. For most people, however, the issue isn't too much exercise but not getting enough. Plus, there are tons of myths about exercise that people subscribe to. Here's the truth behind some common misbeliefs about working out.

- *You Have to Exercise Hard to Get Results*

This is not necessarily true. Moderate aerobic exercise, where you're working hard enough to breathe hard, will convey a slew of health benefits. While interval training is more challenging, the workouts tend to be shorter. When it comes to lifting weights, yes, you want to challenge your muscles beyond what they're used to, but that doesn't mean lifting huge dumbbells. When you slow down and use proper form, you'll be provided with enough of a challenge, and you'll get results.

- *If You Don't Work Out, Muscle Turns to Fat*

Nope. Muscle tissue is muscle tissue, and fat tissue is fat tissue. Yes, former athletes who quit working out may gain body fat, but that's usually due to working out less while eating far more calories than their bodies need. Strength training will help you combat the sarcopenia (loss of muscle) that otherwise occurs in your thirties and older. So, "Use it or lose it."

- *If You Don't Have At Least Thirty Minutes to Exercise, It's Not Worth It*

Slews of studies have shown that short *bursts* of activity (like exercising for five or ten minutes) are as beneficial as longer sessions of exercise. Interestingly, many of the health benefits of exercise, like lowering cholesterol and blood pressure, accrue in the first few minutes of starting to work out. Even a five-minute walk is much better than doing nothing.

- *Lifting Weights Will Give Women Big, Bulky Muscles*

Men and women lose muscle mass at about the same rate in adulthood, but women have less muscle mass in general. The only way to retain that muscle mass is to overload it on a regular basis, such as when you strength train. But women lack the testosterone to build huge muscles. Even most men can't put on muscle without a dedicated program of overloading their bodies and training each muscle group multiple times. Most women notice that they look more toned, their clothes fit better, and it's easier to do everyday tasks when they start lifting weights.

- *Cardio Is the Best Exercise You Can Do*

For years, we've been told that cardio exercise is the answer, but the tide is starting to turn, and now there's more of an emphasis on strength training, especially as you get older. If you only have time to do one form of exercise, I suggest you do strength training. You can accumulate cardio time throughout the day simply by moving more.

- *You Should Exercise the First Thing in the Morning for the Best Results*

There is a kernel of truth to this. People who work out in the morning are more likely to stick with their routines than those who exercise in the afternoon or evening. So, in theory, yes, morning exercisers may reap more health benefits simply because they're sticking with it. But the best time for you to work out is whenever you know you'll be able to do it.

Challenge Your Heart and Lungs: Why Cardio Counts

Strengthening your muscles with moves that challenge them is one part of the *Extinguish the Flame Program* exercise component. The second is to make time for cardiovascular exercise (cardio) several times a week. Cardio activities put sustained demands on your heart and lungs. They include things like walking, biking, swimming, jumping rope, climbing stairs, playing basketball, and tennis. In fact, any activity that gets your heart rate up and keeps it up is cardio, so you have plenty of choices.

Walking is the easiest way to get in a quick session. If you walk fast enough to feel a little out of breath, you're likely at a moderate intensity. A thirty-minute walk several times a week is enough to help combat inflammation, but feel free to swap in other activities so you don't get bored.

To up the ante and reap even more health benefits, you may want to consider interval training. With interval training, you intersperse higher-intensity efforts with recovery instead of maintaining the same intensity. You work harder but for short bursts of time. Because you're working at a higher intensity, you can reap the same fitness benefits in less time, which may reduce your risk of injury as well. You can use any kind of cardio exercise for intervals — walking, stationary biking, or jumping rope, for example.

Here's a walking interval workout to try. Warm up by walking at an easy pace for several minutes. Walk as fast as you can for one minute. You should feel a little breathless. Then, return to your easy pace for one minute. That's one interval, which is also called a 1:1 because your *work* interval is the same as your *rest* interval. Do four to six rounds of this. Then, cool down by walking at an easy pace for three to five minutes. You can make interval workouts more challenging by extending your work intervals, shortening your rest intervals, or doing more intervals in total.

If you haven't tried this type of workout before, pay attention to the way your body feels. You should feel like you're working hard but not like you're about to collapse! Try an interval workout once a week or so for a new challenge and to mix up your routine a little. You may find that you prefer them to be longer and more moderately paced workouts.

> ### *When Too Much Exercise Adds Up:*
> ### *Frank's Story*
>
> Frank, 74, had spent most of his life as an athlete but had suffered a surfing injury a few years earlier. Now, he was in extreme pain due to the injury and was unable to work out, something about which he was passionate.
>
> He'd also been diagnosed with osteoarthritis and said he felt tired, stiff, and tight all over. He was overweight, and his sleep quality was poor. He was waking up several times a night.
>
> Frank was given acupuncture to help his pain, and he increased the amount of water he drank. He also switched to an anti-inflammatory diet that eliminated beer (something he enjoyed), most grains, and sugar. Just as important, he modified his workouts because he was pushing too hard at the gym, causing even more inflammation.
>
> He started taking supplements to help reduce his inflammation, including a green superfood, extracts of turmeric, Boswellia, ginger, and omega-3 fish oil. Digestive supplements and adaptogens were recom-mended to support his gut.
>
> Six months later, his inflammatory markers had improved (C-reactive protein dropped from 3.36 to 1.35, homocysteine from 21.1 to 14.8, and protein-specific antigen, or PSA, from 2.5 to 1.9), and he'd lost 40 pounds

> He was back to his regular workout sessions at the gym, training with guys decades younger than him, started surfing again, and was only getting up once a night instead of five times.
>
> - Chantelle DeShazer, PhD, L.Ac

Cryotherapy

As we mentioned earlier, "Move it or Lose it"! However, when you move your body too much, as in excessive exercise, this can lead to inflammation. Cryotherapy, although not new, has gained much popularity in recent years for its ability to reduce inflammation.

Cryotherapy, a cutting-edge wellness practice, involves exposing the body to extremely low temperatures for short durations, typically ranging from 40°F to 60°F when experiencing an ice bath or cold plunge. Whole-body cryotherapy saunas are powered by either nitrogen or electricity, and the cold air temperature can range from -150-250°F depending on time and cryotherapy brand specifications.

This chilly experience, often referred to as "cold therapy," has gained popularity for its potential health benefits. The primary objective of cryotherapy is to induce a physiological response by exposing the body to intense colds, prompting various reactions that may contribute to improved well-being. Advocates of cryotherapy claim benefits such as reduced muscle soreness, enhanced recovery after physical activity, and potential relief from inflammatory conditions. Dr. Andrew Huberman is a neuroscientist and a professor of neurobiology and ophthalmology at Stanford School of Medicine. He is one of the biggest advocates of cryotherapy and believes, "In the moment if you were to measure somebody's inflammation, you'd say, 'This person is dying. They're in a terrible state.' It's like getting open heart surgery without anesthesia, the way some people react to the ice bath. That really acute adrenaline spike, that pain that you feel creates a higher pain threshold later."

I have personally experienced the benefits of cryotherapy from inflammation resulting from sports activity or working out. I purchased a cold plunge for home use, and in combination with my infrared sauna, it has made a world of difference in reducing inflammation.

Here are some potential health benefits associated with cryotherapy and cold plunge, supported by scientific studies:

- Reduced Inflammation:
    - Cryotherapy, which involves exposure to extremely cold temperatures, has been linked to a reduction in inflammation.

- Pain Relief:
    - Cold exposure has analgesic effects and may contribute to pain relief. Cryotherapy is often used to manage pain associated with conditions like arthritis and muscle injuries.

- Muscle Recovery:
    - Athletes often use cryotherapy for quicker muscle recovery after intense physical activity. The cold temperature may help reduce muscle soreness and enhance recovery.

- Improved Circulation:
    - Cold exposure can stimulate vasoconstriction and vasodilation, potentially leading to improved circulation. This may benefit cardiovascular health and promote better blood flow.

- Boosted Metabolism:
    - Some studies suggest that exposure to cold temperatures can activate brown adipose tissue (BAT), leading to an increase in metabolic rate. This could have implications for weight management.
- Enhanced Mood and Stress Reduction:
    - Cold exposure has been associated with the release of endorphins, contributing to an improved mood. Additionally, it may have stress-reducing effects.
- Skin Health:
    - Cold plunge or cryotherapy sessions may have positive effects on skin health, including increased collagen production and potential benefits for conditions like dermatitis.
- Immune System Modulation:
    - Cold exposure may modulate the immune system, leading to potential benefits in terms of immune function. This can contribute to overall health and well-being.

It's important to note that while these potential benefits are supported by some studies, individual responses to cryotherapy may vary. Always consult with healthcare providers, especially if you have pre-existing health conditions.

Mix up Your Routine: Try an Exercise Class
If you want to stick with a workout plan, enlist a friend to exercise with you. One of the ways to improve exercise adherence, which means your ability to stick with a program, is to work out with someone else. In short, buddying up makes a difference. Talk to a friend, neighbor, or coworker about walking together several times a week, or consider trying an exercise class.

Check out the offerings at your local gym, the Y, or a health club for classes that sound intriguing. Investing in a class makes you more likely to attend, especially if you plan to go with someone else. There's another bonus: You don't have to decide what you'll do that day for a workout. You just show up and follow along with the instructor.

If you're already exercising regularly, taking a class can help you add some variety to your routine. A new class can offer cross-training or exercising in a way you don't usually do it. This can help prevent injury, and it may help reinvigorate a stale routine as well. Look for a class that's different than what you usually do. If you usually swim for exercise, you might try a yoga or weightlifting class. If you always workout inside, you might sign up for a boot camp class that's held outdoors.

Just as important is that a lot of classes are fun! Zumba (a dance class that incorporates upbeat music), indoor cycling, and kickboxing all have their fans. You're likely to push yourself a little harder than you would on your own, and a good instructor will make sure that your form is correct.

If you're nervous about a new class, look for ones that are geared toward beginners, or ask if you can try out a class for free without signing up for the whole session. Most gyms are happy to accommodate this request.

Is Sitting the New Smoking? Move More Often
The third part of the *Extinguish the Flame Program* exercise component is simple, yet most of us fail to do it. It's to add more movement into your day. That's it.

Many people have desk jobs that are literally killing them. Have you heard sitting described as the new smoking? It's that dangerous to your health. Studies show that those who sit for long hours are at greater risk for cancer, heart disease, diabetes (all conditions that are linked with inflammation), and early death. A landmark study published in 2017 found that the more you sit and the longer you sit, the more likely you are to die prematurely, even if you exercise. In other words, that time at the gym won't offset the harmful effect of being nearly motionless the rest of the day.

Let's look at another marker for longevity. A study by Brazilian physician Claudio Gil Soares de Araujo had people between the ages of fifty-one and eighty stand and then sit down on the floor without using hands, knees, or legs for support. This was testing their overall strength and flexibility. In the study, when subjects required more than one hand or knee support to sit and rise from the floor, there was a 2-4-fold higher death rate over a 6.3-year study period.

Wake up! Your body was not designed to sit in a desk chair for eight hours, in a car to drive home, and on a couch for the remainder of the evening while watching brain-draining television, only to crawl into bed exhausted — the quintessential couch potato.

Just stop. We are killing ourselves with sitting and sedentary lifestyles. If not our bodies, we're certainly killing our spirits. Have you seen the movie *WALL-E*? We are moving toward becoming those people-shaped blobs that ride around on robots and stare at screens all day. If you don't believe me, just look at all of the technology that offers alternatives to walking. I'm not talking about automobiles or motorcycles. I'm talking about things like motorized Segways, E-bikes, hoverboards, and yet another way to be despicably lazy, the UNI-CUB personal transporter, which requires even less effort than the others, as you are literally sitting while riding. At least with bicycles, skateboards, and inline skates, body mechanics and exertion are involved).

I acknowledge the innovation of these products and the fact that they are helping some of the population with disabilities who can't get around that easily. Sadly, people who are perfectly capable of walking are also using them instead of using their legs.

So, what's the answer? Reject the technology that's designed to help you be lazy and make a concerted, intentional effort to get out of your chair and move more. Your goal should be to get up at least every hour. Even better is moving every thirty minutes. This may not be possible during an hour-long commute to work, so look for times when you can either sit less, move more, or both.

Sit Less and Move More
It's easy to forget how long you've been sitting if you're engrossed in work. Set a timer on your watch or computer to remind you to get up and stretch or walk up and down the hallway for a couple of minutes. Make it a habit to stand up whenever you answer your phone or receive a text (You may also realize how much time — possibly too much time — you spend texting).

At work, break up meetings by suggesting a stretching break every hour or so. Better yet, try a walking meeting. You can dictate notes on your smartphone using an app. Standing desks are gaining popularity. If you don't have one, try putting your laptop or computer in a box on your desk. Just make sure that you can type comfortably in this position.

We've gotten used to taking shortcuts, so try the opposite approach. Instead of looking for the closest parking spot to your destination, park farther away and walk the difference. If you take public transportation, get off at an earlier stop and walk the remainder of the way. Take a couple of laps around the perimeter of the grocery store before you start shopping. Take the stairs instead of the elevator. Simply wearing a Fitbit or having another fitness app can motivate you to walk more. See the following section titled "Can a Bracelet Make You Fitter?"

Household chores count as movement, too. Tasks like sweeping, vacuuming, dusting, doing laundry, and washing dishes all keep you moving. Work in your yard or garden or tackle that household task (like finally painting the guest room) instead of hiring someone to do it.

Even if you're active during the day, you may spend a lot of time sitting at night. If you're watching television, get up during every set of commercials, even if it's just to stretch for a minute or two. Try taking a short walk or bike ride after dinner. It's a nice way to unwind after a meal and can double as quality time with your mate or family.

Can a Bracelet Make You Fitter?
The Secret to Walking More

Chances are that you know someone who sports a Fitbit, Apple watch, or other wearable technology that measures how active that person is. If you want to become more active, simply wearing a device like this can help.

An interesting study published in 2007 found that people who were asked to wear a pedometer and track how many steps they took each day averaged more than two thousand extra steps per day — that's about an extra mile of walking. Another more recent study included 142 adults who were asked to walk 10,000 steps per day and to wear pedometers to track their progress.

Participants walked about 10,700 steps per day during the first month and averaged 6,300 steps by the end of the sixth month, but they were still more active than they had been originally. They had reduced their overall belly fat without changing their diets.

The average adult walks between two-and-a-half-to-three miles a day, which is the equivalent of five thousand to six thousand steps. That's just half of the suggested ten thousand steps per day that are supposed to promote good health. By the way, there's no *official* ten thousand steps recommendation. The guideline is based on research that shows the healthiest adults walk quite a bit — between seven thousand and thirteen thousand steps a day.

You needn't invest in a Fitbit. An inexpensive pedometer that you clip on your clothes will work just fine. Set a baseline of how many steps you average. It may be much lower than you expected. Then, set a goal of walking more, like adding two thousand steps a day or an additional mile of walking. At a brisk pace, you should cover about 1.5 to 2 miles in thirty to forty-five minutes of walking. It may take a while to achieve this pace, but stick with it, and you'll be surprised at how soon you'll be walking at this speed.

The elements of this step aren't complicated, but I realize that many people have trouble starting or sticking with an exercise routine. What's my best advice? Stop thinking of moving more as something you *have* to do and look for activities you enjoy, whether that's yoga, a cycling class, or walking with a neighbor several mornings a week. The more pleasure you find in the activity, the more likely you are to continue it.

If your schedule doesn't allow you to stay with a dedicated workout plan, simply make sure that you're up and moving as often as you can during the day. That's a habit that may be easier to maintain, which means that it's even better for fighting inflammation in the long run.

Chapter 8
Stress Less

Step Four of the Extinguish the Flame Program

Play is where the mind, body, and spirit unite as one for the sole purpose of enjoyment.

- Bruce Howe, DC, CCN, author

In the last chapter, you learned that you're more likely to stick with any kind of exercise if you enjoy it. That makes sense, right? The idea of finding pleasure in working out may be a stretch for you, but it's a logical transition into the fourth step of the *Extinguish the Flame Program*, which includes adding more play into your life and better-managing stressors.

Some stress is inescapable. Everyone faces financial worries, health concerns, or family drama, at least some of the time. However, what matters isn't the stress but the way you respond to it. When you add more health-enhancing activities to your life, things like playing more, laughing more frequently, expressing love, and embracing gratitude, you're better equipped to handle stress. In other words, stress has less of an impact on you, and it is less likely to fuel inflammation.

Play More: The Missing Element of Health
Play is, perhaps, one of the most neglected elements of a healthy lifestyle. Play is the place where mind, body, and spirit unite. God created this beautiful planet as a playground for us to enjoy His creation, but often, we are so caught up

in the busyness of life that we forget to enjoy it. Play is the catalyst for joy. This space allows us to "live deep and suck out all the marrow of life," as author Henry David Thoreau wrote in his famous book *On Walden Pond*. Playing and enjoying life is where we find meaning, connection, and vitality. Only from this place of joyful expression and connection can we truly create and live out our purpose, do our best work, be fully expressed, and be our best selves.

Play can be anything: laughing, exploring, dancing, singing, painting, writing, cycling, gaming, riding, running, walking, or gardening. It can be your favorite sport: volleyball, basketball, tennis, baseball, football, wrestling, martial arts, soccer, pickleball, or track and field. Play is hide-and-seek in the neighborhood, stealing time by the creek in the afternoon, catching fireflies on a summer's evening, freeze tag in the backyard, and picnics in the park.

It's composing poetry, snapping breathtaking photographs, hosting a dinner party, celebrating a promotion, or surprising someone on his or her birthday. It's stargazing with your beloved, tending to a garden, hiking a mountain with your best friend, playing music, and rearranging your furniture. It's walking dogs for the local animal shelter or volunteering and spending time as a Big Brother or Big Sister. It's kayaking down the river, discovering a new golf swing, diving into a new swimming hole, snorkeling along a reef, walking down the beach at sunset, or making love to your spouse. It's whatever lights you up! Have I inspired you yet?

Play not only gives pleasure but is also one of the most effective stress relievers. When you're playing, you're caught up in what you're doing. You're free from the worries of your work, family, health, or future. Play lets you enter a state of *flow*, which is a highly focused mental state where you lose track of time. Flow can occur during any kind of play or activity that requires concentration. If you've ever lost track of time while pursuing a hobby, laughing with a friend, or even strolling in a beautiful park, you've likely experienced flow.

Play isn't only for vacation time. It is meant for everyday life. But when it comes to vacations, Americans are notoriously the worst at taking them. Our nation is the only Westernized country that does not have any mandatory or legally required vacation days or holidays. Compare this to European countries where employers are required by law to give a minimum of four weeks' worth of vacation time. Austria and Portugal give employees a mandatory thirty-five days off per year. Germany and Spain are just behind them with thirty-four days per year. France gives thirty-one days off per year. Employees in Belgium, Italy, and New Zealand have thirty days off per year.

How is it that our country, which is supposed to be so progressive, doesn't understand the value of time off for well-being? It even says in our Declaration of Independence that we, as Americans, have the right to the "pursuit of happiness." When, exactly, are we supposed to pursue said happiness? It doesn't all have to be work, work, work, even in America. Yet the average employer only offers two weeks' vacation, and many workers don't even take all of their vacation days.

So, when was the last time you played? I mean, *really* played and enjoyed yourself? Recently, I hope. If not, why not? Perhaps your job demands all of your time and energy. That's understandable. Is there any way you can bring some element of play into your workday? Even taking five minutes here and there to walk around outside, bounce a ball, jump rope, or get some fresh air can lighten your spirit and restore a little vitality. I hope you're one who finds time to play every single day. If you're really, *really* lucky, you get to thoroughly enjoy whatever it is you're doing while you're working.

Consider what Francois Auguste Rene de Chateaubriand, a French writer and diplomat, said.

A master in the art of living draws no sharp distinction between his work and his play, his labor and his leisure, his mind and his body, his education and his recreation. He hardly knows which is which. He simply pursues his vision of excellence through whatever he is doing and leaves others to determine whether he is working or playing. To himself, he always appears to be doing both.

I realize that this may be a tall order for many people. So, start by adding play to your life in small doses, if necessary.

A word of caution to those who are pursuing athletic endeavors: While moderate exercise fights inflammation, it's possible to overdo it, especially if you have a sedentary job and work out sporadically. Some people save up all of their playtime for the weekends and go a little too hard to make up for lost time. These weekend warriors are more likely to overexert themselves, which may result in an ankle sprain during soccer, a torn hamstring during a pickup basketball game, or shin splints from a long run. You may be striving to get rid of some stress or engaging in friendly competition without realizing that you're setting yourself up for injury. This has never been more evident than with the phenomenal growth of pickleball. Now the fastest growing sport in America. Doctors and therapists are treating more injuries from pickleball than any other sport.

I speak from experience. Now that I'm in my seventies, I've had to be mindful of what my body can and can't do. Sometimes, I think I'm still twenty. Many men are like that. The testosterone kicks in, and we think we can still do what we did twenty, thirty, or forty years ago. Maybe we can — until we blow out a knee or strain a shoulder.

The key is to find that sweet spot between being a weekend warrior and a couch potato, where you're playing, laughing, and engaging in regular physical activity as often as you can in order to have a healthy mind-body-spirit balance.

Consider these questions to help you add more play to your life.

- What did you enjoy doing as a child?
- What do you enjoy doing now?
- When are you the happiest?
- What makes you laugh? (We'll talk more about laughter in the next section).
- When was the last time you *really* laughed?
- Whom do you love being around?
- Which people in your life inspire you to play?
- How can you fit more play into your day?
- What are your favorite physical activities or sports?

Put Play into Action: Fifteen Ideas for More Fun

Do you still need some playful ideas? Here are fifteen activities you may enjoy.

1. Host a game night or a dinner party with your favorite people.
2. Join a local sports league to play softball, volleyball, soccer, pickleball, or tennis.
3. Attend a live music event.
4. Try an activity you've never done before, like kayaking, snowboarding, zip-lining, or stand-up paddle boarding.
5. Take music lessons.
6. Attend a stand-up comedy show.
7. Check out www.Meetup.com for a list of events, activities, and groups in your city or neighborhood.

There is a meetup for nearly every interest you can imagine. Whether you're into food, sports, knitting, golf, music, gaming, movies, or books, you'll probably find something that appeals to you.
8. Are you a treasure hunter at heart? Try geocaching, where you learn the online coordinates for thousands of hidden treasures throughout the world and then go on foot to find them. When you do find one, take out the treasure and put one of your own inside (Check out www.geocaching.com for more info).
9. If you enjoy the outdoors, explore a local trail, mountain, cave, or park.
10. If the wilderness isn't your thing, try an urban hike. You can create your own theme. Instead of a pub crawl, you might try a foodie crawl where you start with a light breakfast at one end of town, have a vibrant green juice in another part of town, or a glass of wine or ice cold beer (remember to limit it to one), and end with a healthy dinner in yet another part of town, all the while exploring and playing in your city. Some other ideas would be a museum crawl, coffee/tea crawl, a historical walking tour, a haunted tour, or anything else that excites you).
11. If you're a shutterbug, grab your camera, explore, and create art along the way.
12. Take dance lessons.
13. Go dancing and show off your new moves.
14. Join a book or movie club or start your own with some friends.
15. Do something that scares you a little bit. (Karaoke, maybe?)

Come on. You only live once!

Laugh More: A Proven Stress-Buster
Laughter truly is one of the best medicines, yet the older you are, the less likely you are to laugh. Research reveals that

children laugh about two hundred to three hundred times a day, while adults laugh on average only fifteen to twenty times. Adults should be laughing more — much more.

Don't confuse humor with laughter. Humor is a cognitive stimulus or something that our brains may interpret as funny or amusing. Laughter is a psychophysiological response. This is where the magic happens. Laughing changes your body's chemistry. It immediately lowers your blood pressure, suppresses the stress hormone cortisol (the major stress hormone), and triggers the release of serotonin (a brain chemical that produces a feeling of relaxation and is sometimes called the happy hormone) and endorphins, (pain-killing, feel-good chemicals).

Studies examining laughter's impact on health have found that even a brief period of laughter boosts immune function. It also improves mood and eases anxiety. Laughter engages the diaphragm and stimulates the vagus nerve (the longest nerve of the autonomic nervous system). This nerve is a key to the brain-body connection and communicates messages between the gut and the brain and the heart and the brain. Stimulating it seems to tell your body to relax.

Laughter temporarily takes our minds off our troubles and shuts off the constant inner mental chatter we all experience. For another way to turn off that chatter, see the next section on becoming more mindful. More laughter means you're taking in more oxygen and releasing oxytocin (the *really* good feeling hormone associated with love). More of these two *oxy* elements means that you have healthier lungs, a sharper mind, and more of the good chemicals to fight against any physical and mental stressors.

So, this is all good news. What's surprising is that you don't have to actually laugh for health benefits. Even fake laughter changes your body chemistry. One study found that adults who forced themselves to laugh for just one minute improved their moods. Sometimes, fake laughter turns into the real thing. Try fake laughing with a friend. Chances are that you'll start to genuinely crack up.

To add more laughter to your life, give these strategies a try.

- *What Do You Find Funny?*

Whether it's a favorite sitcom, playing with your cat or dog, or calling one of your entertaining friends, identify your own *laughter buttons* and push them frequently.

- *Start Laughter Library*

This might include authors you find amusing, bookmarked websites that crack you up, or YouTube channels that feature your favorite comedians or silly cat videos. Do whatever works for you.

- *Spend More Time with People You Enjoy*

Hey, not everyone is funny, but chances are that you have at least one or two people in your life who can make you laugh.

- *Look For the Absurdities in Life*

If you look for humor in your everyday life, you're likely to find it.

Becoming More Mindful: Slowing Down the Monkey Mind

Close your eyes for a few seconds. Let your mind wander. What's going on in your head? If you're like most of us, you've got what seems like a million thoughts racing through your mind at any given moment. Becoming mindful is shorthand for slowing down, becoming aware of what's happening in the present, and embracing the now instead of regretting the past or worrying about the future. You simply "Focus on the moment. Stay in the moment." as the saying goes — Tony Horton.

Research suggests that mindfulness practices like meditation may ease anxiety and depression and help you cope with stress better. Taking time to practice being mindful may also make it easier to learn, concentrate, manage your emotions, and improve your outlook. It's also a way of giving your brain a break.

It's simple to do. Take a couple of minutes to ground yourself. Become aware of what's around you. What do you see? What do you hear or smell? What's happening around you? What sensations do you have in your body?

Focus on your breathing. Take some slow, deep inhalations and exhalations. Notice how that produces a sense of relaxation. As thoughts cross your mind, simply notice them and move on.

Taking a few moments to stop, focus, and re-center yourself can help you shake off stress and reset yourself, even in the middle of the busiest day.

Love More: People Matter Most

Mahatma Gandhi once said, "Where there is love, there is life." Without love, can life really have meaning?

Love plays a role in overall health, and it can have a powerful impact on healing. For example, one study found that both men and women who were married were 2.5 times more likely to be alive fifteen years after coronary-artery-bypass grafting (major surgery to treat heart disease) than those who were not married. Even more significantly, those who were the happiest with their marriages were the most likely to be alive.

It's not just your romantic relationships that impact your health. A review study published in 2013 found that the quality of a person's relationships with his or her family members, friends, and spouse affected that person's risk of developing depression. People who said that they had the lowest-quality relationships were more than twice as likely to become depressed as those people who were the most satisfied with theirs.

Love can ward off depression, which may help to fight off inflammation. In fact, depression can actually *contribute* to inflammation. Studies have found that inflammation and depression fuel each other. Inflammation can contribute to depression in some people. Depression may also affect your gut health — the microbiome — causing inflammation. Interestingly, the research suggests a link between the two: Treating one may help improve the other.

The physical expression of affection can also affect your health. Holding hands or being touched by someone you love reduces anxiety and the perception of pain and improves your mood. It works with animals, too. Stroking a cat or dog immediately lowers blood pressure and heart rate. A review study on the impact of touch therapy, which can include anything from a hug to a massage, on people with cancer found that touch can help ease nausea, pain, anxiety, and fatigue, as well as improve overall quality of life.

You have people in your life whom you love. You have things you love to do. Focusing on them can help heal your mind, body, and spirit. When you are in love (the act of loving yourself and others), you heal your brain and flood your body with all of the good chemicals it needs to be full of vitality. That makes you more resistant to inflammation.

This is just a reminder, or perhaps a wake-up call, not only to put a little love in your heart but also to express it. People who are more affectionate bounce back from stress more quickly, are less likely to be depressed, sleep better, and have better immune function than those who aren't as quick to share their feelings.

Here are four easy ways to express love:

- *Use Touch to Connect*

A hug, a gentle squeeze of the arm, and even a brief peck on the cheek all trigger the release of oxytocin, the powerful feel-good chemical. It is sometimes referred to as the love hormone because levels of oxytocin increase during hugging and sexual intimacy. It may benefit people suffering from conditions such as depression, anxiety, and intestinal problems.

- *Make Time for the People Who Matter*

You must spend many of your waking hours at work, but don't become so career-focused that you lose sight of what's really important: the people in your life. Spend quality time with them.

- *Stay Connected with Far-Flung Family Members and Friends*

Take advantage of technology to keep in touch with your kids, grandkids, friends, and other family members. Text, email, Skype, Zoom, call — whatever helps you maintain that connection even long distance. Don't overlook handwritten notes and letters.

- *Put It in Writing*

Interesting research shows that simply writing down what you love about someone improves your mood and outlook. Focusing on the positives about someone else is likely to improve your relationship, too.

Be Grateful: Beyond Saying Thanks

We've talked about several powerful ways to combat stress. There's one more thing that is amazingly simple yet effective: Practice gratitude on a regular basis.

Robert Emmons, PhD, the leading gratitude researcher and a professor of psychology at the University of California/Davis, suggests that being grateful is actually a two-step process. First, you recognize what is good about your life.

Second, you acknowledge that goodness comes not from you but from someone else, whether that's God, another person, or even an animal.

> One of Emmons's best-known studies divided college students into three groups. Each was asked to list five things that had happened during the prior week. One group listed five things that had occurred, one group listed five things that had upset or annoyed them, and one group listed five things that they were grateful for. Ten weeks later, the *grateful group* reported having more optimism. They slept better and even had fewer colds than the other two groups of students. What's the takeaway? Gratitude appears to boost immune function.

Expressing gratitude makes you more likely to feel happiness, enthusiasm, joy, love, and optimism and less likely to experience feelings like envy, resentment, and bitterness. Gratitude also makes you more resilient to daily stressors.

Yet just as we fail to take vacation time, Americans as a whole tend to come up short on gratitude. We're surrounded by a culture that is focused on getting *more* — more money, more success, more possessions, and more toys — instead of focusing on having what we want and wanting what we have. But with practice, being grateful is easier than you might think.

Try these techniques to embrace more thankfulness.

- *Keep a Gratitude Journal*

At the end of the day, write down three things that you're grateful for. It could be as small as the fact that it was a warm, sunny day, that your body feels good, or that you enjoyed a healthy lunch outside during your lunch break. Studies show this simple exercise (counting three of your blessings) every day can lower your risk of depression and make you happier.

- *Pray*

If you believe in a higher power, take the time to thank God for the world in which you live, for your body, for waking up to another day, and for the people in your life. Prayer is often about requesting help instead of simply being grateful for all that you've been given. Remedy that.

- *Thank Someone in Writing*

When was the last time you got a thankyou note? They may be rare these days, but why not take the time to thank someone who has made a difference in your life?

Maybe it was a teacher, a coach, a boss, a neighbor, or a friend who helped you through a tough time. Tell the person how he or she impacted your life and the reason that you appreciate it. You may even make this a weekly habit.

- *Volunteer*

Helping someone else is one way to express gratitude, and it helps make the world a better place.

- *Make It a Habit*

On a day when everything's going well, it's easy to be grateful. Some days it's harder. When you practice gratitude on a regular basis, you'll find that it is easier to focus on what you already have and find that everyday annoyances don't bother you quite as much.

- *Reframe Your Thinking*

Years ago, actress Jamie Lee Curtis said during an interview that she tries not to say, "I have to." For example, "I have to go grocery shopping." She says, "I get to." "I get to go grocery shopping." After all, you are physically able to go to the store, and you can afford to buy food for yourself and your family. This simple reframing can make you aware of how much you tend to take for granted.

Do you know anyone who seems grateful for just about everything or someone who's relentlessly positive? After a breakup, your sister might say, "Well, I'd rather have loved and lost than never have loved at all." Your friend gets fired, and he says, "I know there's a better job out there for me. Now I can take a vacation." Your neighbor has to relocate for work and insists it's an opportunity for a new adventure.

This kind of Pollyanna attitude can be annoying at times, but being grateful for even the challenges that you face makes you happier. It makes you more resistant to stress, which means you're more resistant to inflammation as well. If you tend to see the glass as half-empty instead of half-full, or you know that you usually look at the negative side of things, try looking deeper to see if you can discover the blessings in your circumstances. It takes practice, but with time, it will become a healthy and gratifying habit.

Keeping Stress from Stressing You Out
Stress may be inescapable, but you can make your body and brain more resilient to it. Loving, laughing, playing — this is the stuff of life!

Not only will embracing the strategies in this chapter fight inflammation, but they'll also bring more joy, satisfaction, and happiness to your life. Consider this as your permission and prescription to have more fun.

Chapter 9
Better Sleep, Better Health

Step Five of the Extinguish the Flame Program

Sleep is that golden chain that ties health and our bodies together.

- Thomas Dekker, English dramatist

Americans are not only vacation-deprived and fun-deprived but also sleep-deprived. We routinely sacrifice sleep to catch up on work, socialize, or simply watch television, but all of that sleep debt adds up. The connection between sleep and inflammation is well documented. Studies show shorting yourself on as little as a couple of hours a night (sleeping only five hours instead of your usual seven, for example) alters markers of inflammation. The less quality sleep you get, the more dramatic an impact it may have on your body.

Sleep has long been both a personal and professional interest of mine. My older brother, Dr. Maynard Howe, was diagnosed with a learning disability at age thirteen because he had been constantly falling asleep in class. Because of his inability to concentrate and his consequent poor grades, he was placed in a class for slow learners.

He was nineteen years old when he discovered that his battle with allergies was contributing to his lack of sleep and concentration. When he moved from the environment that was contributing to his allergies and made some dietary changes, he realized that he didn't have a learning disability. His sleep habits improved as well. That was a real eye-opener for Maynard. He eventually graduated cum laude with a PhD in psychology.

Maynard's experience was the catalyst for my interest in sleep. Over the years, I have come to appreciate the profound effect that changing your diet and making other lifestyle modifications can have on sleep quality.

In short, better nutrition leads to better sleep, which leads to better health. But the converse is also true. Better nutrition makes for better health, which makes for better sleep. It's tied together. It's difficult to determine whether it's sleep or diet — which is the chicken and which is the egg. They work together.

Running on Empty: Why Sleep Is So Important

Sleep does more than provide a bridge from one day to the next. It's when your body does most of its healing and the repair of your tissues and organs. This is critical for immune function. An ongoing lack of sleep is linked to inflammation, and it puts you at higher risk of diseases, including heart disease, stroke, diabetes, and high blood pressure.

Sleep also has a powerful impact on how well your brain functions. Quality sleep helps you learn new skills, remember information, and pay attention. When you're short on sleep, you may have trouble making decisions and controlling your emotions. You won't be as productive at work. Worst of all, just a few hours of lost sleep can impact you as dramatically as if you hadn't slept at all!

Going into nocturnal overdrive to get a job done or hang out with friends may seem harmless, but you could be sacrificing your health if you do it regularly. The body identifies a lack of sleep as a state of stress. Once in stress mode, your body responds by raising levels of stress hormones like adrenaline and cortisol. Hormones regulate functions like blood pressure and insulin levels, and when you're in a constant state of stress, these levels can be difficult to control. Your immune system also becomes impaired.

Even mild sleep deprivation disrupts the normal levels of the hormones ghrelin and leptin, which regulate appetite. Low levels of leptin can make you crave carbs and high-sugar foods and overeat. Studies show that those who sleep the least are more prone to gain weight than those who get more sack time.

If you wake frequently during the night, you may never get into deep REM (rapid eye movement) sleep. REM sleep is important because it is the restorative part of your sleep cycle. It also stimulates the regions of the brain that are used in learning and memory.

Even short periods of sleep deprivation can affect every system of your body and lead to

- blurry vision
- cognitive impairment
- depression
- hallucinations and psychosis (with long-term sleep deprivation)
- headaches
- heart palpitations
- hyperactivity
- impaired immune system
- increased blood pressure
- irritability
- memory lapses
- muscle aches
- under-eye circles
- weight gain or loss (although it's usually gain)

Usually, the symptoms of short-term sleep deprivation can be reversed by getting the proper amount of sleep right away. If you've tried to sleep, and you are still waking up exhausted, you may have a medical condition like sleep apnea (more about those in a bit). Consult with your physician for testing and evaluation.

The Eight-Hour Myth: How Much Sleep Do You Need?
So, how much sleep do you need to function at your best? Eight hours may be the recommended amount for most adults, but the *amount* of sleep may not be as important as the *quality* of that sleep. Working with patients, I've found quality depends on many factors, including diet and — you guessed it — inflammation. The bottom line is that many people sleep poorly, and they may not even realize how fragmented their sleep is until it improves and they feel significantly better.

The cause of sleeplessness is a multifactorial issue. People are undernourished and over-caffeinated (Caffeine is perhaps the biggest culprit to sleepless nights). Many of us stay connected to screens of some sort (televisions, computers, electronic tablets, and smartphones), watching movies, playing video games, or checking social media right up until we go to bed. Daily stress, especially if you don't exercise, also contributes to poor sleep.

So what's the answer? First, set the stage for restful sleep. If you make sleep a priority and create a sleep-conducive environment but still feel tired every morning, you may have a sleep-related disorder. You'll learn more about common disorders and the way to treat them later in this chapter.

Sleep Time Recommendations: What's Changed?
"The NSF has committed to regularly reviewing and providing scientifically rigorous recommendations," says Max Hirshkowitz, PhD, chair of the National Sleep Foundation Scientific Advisory Council. "The public can be confident that these recommendations represent the best guidance for sleep duration and health."

A new range has been added to acknowledge the individual variability in appropriate sleep durations. The recommendations now define times as either

    a. recommended
    b. may be appropriate for some individuals

c. not recommended

The panel revised the recommended sleep ranges for all six children and teenage groups. A summary of the new recommendations includes

- Newborns (0–3 months): Sleep range narrowed to 14–17 hours each day (previously was 12–18)
- Infants (4–11 months): Sleep range widened by 2 hours to 12–15 hours (previously was 14–15)
- Toddlers (1–2 years): Sleep range widened by 1 hour to 11–14 hours (previously was 12–14)
- Preschoolers (3–5 years): Sleep range widened by 1 hour to 10–13 hours (previously was 11–13)
- School-age children (6–13 years): Sleep range widened by 1 hour to 9–11 hours (previously was 10–11)
- Teenagers (14–17 years): Sleep range widened by 1 hour to 8–10 hours (previously was 8.5–9.5)
- Young adults (18–25): Sleep range is 7–9 hours (new age category)
- Adults (26–64): Sleep range did not change and remains 7–9 hours.
- Older adults (65+): Sleep range is 7–8 hours (new age category)

In Search of Slumber: How to Sleep Better Every Night
So, now that you know the importance of sleep to your overall physical and psychological health, let's talk about how to help you and your family sleep better.

- *Set the Stage for Sleep*

Make your room dark, quiet, and cool (Between sixty-eight and seventy degrees is the most conducive to sleep). A bedroom environment that supports uninterrupted rest will leave you feeling more refreshed the next morning and will improve the quality of your REM sleep.

- *Remove Light Sources from Your Bedroom*

Your bedroom is likely brighter than you realize. Many of us have a night light or a clock on the nightstand, and streetlights hold vigil until dawn. But that light can trick your brain into thinking that it's daytime. According to the American Academy of Sleep Medicine, too much light can produce non-restorative, poor-quality sleep.

For deeper sleep, mimic the light-dark cycles of nature by shutting off all lights and using curtains or shades to block outside light sources. Having your alarm clock within view can lead to anxiety and sleeplessness, especially if you have insomnia, so it's best to turn it away from you.

- *Eliminate Sound*

Make your bedroom a sanctuary for resting by eliminating disturbances from computer fans, pets, leaky faucets, or loud music. Clearing your space of *noise clutter* will go a long way in providing better sleep on a regular basis. If you share a room with a snorer or live in a busy neighborhood, consider using earplugs, a noise-canceling machine, or a fan. The gentle sound generated by a white-noise machine or fan can mask low to moderate noises, while earplugs can help block noisy distractions. Earplugs also let you focus on the sound of your breathing and heartbeat, which may help you fall asleep faster.

- *Avoid Alcohol*

Although alcohol may decrease the time it takes to fall asleep, it has the opposite effect on the duration of sleep, especially if you have more than one drink close to bedtime. According to the National Institute on Alcohol Abuse and Alcoholism, consuming just one drink within six hours of bedtime can affect the second stage of sleep by increasing wakefulness, which can make it difficult to fall back asleep if you awaken. This fragmented sleep pattern prevents you from getting sufficient REM sleep and the rest you need.

- *Avoid Caffeine and Nicotine*

Even a small amount of caffeine increases wakefulness, and too much can cause insomnia, jitters, headaches, irregular heartbeat, racing heart, and anxiety. If you drink coffee or tea, have your last cup by early afternoon to give your body a chance to eliminate the caffeine. Make sure that you're not consuming caffeine from other sources (like chocolate) close to bedtime. Cigarettes and other tobacco products also inhibit sleep (See the following section titled "The 'Relaxing' Cigarette: Debunking the Myth").

The "Relaxing" Cigarette: Debunking the Myth

Do you think that an evening cigarette will help you relax? The illusion that a cigarette has a calming effect is false. In fact, the nicotine in tobacco is a stimulant that is likely to keep you awake. The relaxation that a smoker feels when he lights up is the effect of dopamine being released. Within ten seconds of inhaling nicotine, it enters the bloodstream and acts upon the brain cells.

Molecules of nicotine fit like keys into nicotinic receptors on the brain's neurons. These keys fit into the same neurotransmitters as acetylcholine, which plays an important role in alertness, attention, and sensory perception. This reaction causes acetylcholine to overwork, but it's short-lived. Within 30 to 120 minutes after having a cigarette, the nicotine level in the brain drops, and the smoker feels tired and sluggish. The smoker then craves another cigarette, starting the cycle again.

So, that late-night cigarette may leave you revved up rather than relaxed. Smoking may also increase the risk of sleep disorders like obstructive sleep apnea. For better sleep and better health, consider giving up nicotine for good.

- *Leave the Baggage outside of the Bedroom*

Seventy percent of Americans say that they are affected by stress or anxiety every day, which often leads to difficulty sleeping. These stress-induced sleep problems increase as your stress levels increase.

In our multitasking world, you may have to train yourself to let go of your worries at bedtime so that you can sleep better. Try to consciously clear your mind of clutter when you get into bed. Let go of the chatter and remind yourself that you can solve the problem tomorrow.

You can also try keeping a journal. Before bedtime, write about your worries *as if they were already solved.* You don't have to detail how that happened, but only that they *are* resolved and that you're enjoying the harmony of its results. The feeling of thankfulness will go a long way in helping you relax and get into better sleep.

- *Create a Bedtime Routine*

A routine sleep-wake pattern will help ensure that you get optimal sleep most nights. Your brain has a circadian rhythm that serves as an internal body clock. Regular sleep patterns strengthen this inner clock and help you function better.

- *Clear the Clutter*

Is your bedroom a calming or crowded place? Put away clothes, clear away clutter, and eliminate objects that may distract or overstimulate your mind before bedtime.

- *Eliminate Electronics*

Research shows that the blue light emitted from cell phones, computer screens, and televisions interrupts the body's natural rhythms, making the body think it is daytime. This inhibits the production of melatonin, the sleep hormone, and keeps you awake. Consider making your bedroom a tech-free zone because it can be too tempting to check your phone if it buzzes in the middle of the night. This tech tapping disrupts sleep and makes it harder to fall back to sleep.

- *Relax*

Maybe you need a warm Epsom salt bath. Topical applications of lavender oil can be very calming. Try reading before bedtime or some gentle stretching. Choose something that helps you wind down before bed. Late-night business calls, loud music, and to-do lists are counterproductive to relaxation. Instead, consider an evening restorative yoga class, an audiobook, a fireside chat, a relaxation CD, listening to calming music, doing a peaceful visualization meditation, or creating a bedtime tea ceremony as part of your winding-down routine. Have fun creating a ritual that works for you and leaves you feeling relaxed and ready for a good night's sleep.

- *Invest in a High-Quality Mattress*

What's the most used piece of furniture in your home? Your mattress is. You spend six to nine hours on it per night, so it's wise to spend time investigating what's inside your mattress as well as what it feels like when you lie on it. The best mattresses will keep your spine in alignment regardless of your sleeping position.

- *Consider Supplements*

Certain supplements can help you sleep better. Taking magnesium, a natural muscle relaxant, can help you fall asleep faster. An amino acid called L-theanine, which is in green tea, can also help ease you into sleep. Try taking it within fifteen to twenty minutes prior to going to bed. The amino acid 5-HTP, a precursor to tryptophan, increases serotonin (the good-mood chemical), which may also help you slip into sleep. Certain botanical supplements, such as passion flower, hops, valerian root, and lemon balm, have all been shown to be beneficial for the reduction of stress and improving sleep. Passion-flower contains the highest level of GABA or gamma-aminobutyric acid. GABA calms nerve activity in the brain and helps to promote the onset of sleep and maintain its duration. Make sure to look for extracts of these botanicals, as they will yield the highest level of active ingredients for the best results.

CBD, CBN, and Cannabidiols from cannabis are newcomers on the scene and are beneficial for some with sleep disorders. However, it's not legal in all states, and a prescription may be required for it, so check with your local authorities about availability. Finally, a dose of melatonin helps some people sleep. Talk to your healthcare provider about the proper dosage.

When You Still Can't Sleep: Sleep Disorders and Ways to Treat Them

If you've followed the above advice and still can't sleep, you may have a sleep disorder. Treating it can help you achieve the sleep your body and brain need.

- *Insomnia*

It's normal to sleep poorly once in a while. If it occurs several times a week, however, you may be among the sixty million Americans who suffer from insomnia.

A major cause of insomnia is the stress that most of us are subject to on a daily basis. The biochemical survival response that enables you to avoid an oncoming car or juggle your finances when you have more bills than you do paycheck is not meant to be revved up 24-7. Demands come at us from voicemails, cell phones, text messages, computers, and emails. In our hyper-connected society, we're exposed to them nearly all the time. Left unchecked, the deluge of demands can make it all but impossible to relax in the evening.

Other causes of insomnia include depression and anxiety, both of which can interfere with sleep. As you just learned, things like caffeine, nicotine, and alcohol can contribute to insomnia. Certain prescription medications, including sedatives, and medical conditions like chronic pain can contribute as well.

Common signs of insomnia include lying awake for forty-five minutes or longer before falling asleep, sleeping for only short periods, waking frequently, being awake much of the night, and feeling exhausted in the morning. You may feel irritable, have trouble focusing, or have frequent headaches and gastrointestinal issues. Continued insomnia can lead to anxiety, depression, and worries about your sleeplessness, which can make insomnia even worse.

To treat insomnia, try following the guidelines for better sleep provided earlier in this chapter. If it continues to be an issue and you're getting six or fewer hours of sleep per night at least three or four times a week, talk to your doctor about ways to treat it. You may be referred to a sleep center for special testing and diagnostics.

- *Snoring*

About thirty million Americans snore. You're more likely to snore if you're overweight, if you have allergies, a cold, or flu symptoms, and if you smoke or are exposed to second-hand smoke.

If your partner's snoring is keeping you up, the most cost-effective solution is to use earplugs. You can also try a white-noise machine, which can help mask snoring.

If you're the one who snores, try changing positions. Sleeping on your side should help. Avoid alcoholic beverages before bedtime because they can relax your airway muscles and cause snoring (Sleeping pills can have the same effect). Other remedies include certain types of pillows, chinstraps, sprays, nasal strips, mouthpieces, and more. The vast number of choices can be perplexing. You can even sew tennis balls into the back of your pajamas to prevent you from sleeping on your back.

There are plenty of inexpensive anti-snoring devices out there. If you've tried them and snoring is still an issue, talk to your doctor about whether an evaluation at a sleep center is appropriate. Loud or chronic snoring can indicate sleep apnea. Your doctor may also recommend an FDA–approved procedure called somnoplasty to reduce snoring.

- *Sleep Apnea*

The word *apnea* is Greek for *without breath*. If you have sleep apnea, you stop breathing for at least ten seconds at a time before gasping for breath, which dramatically impacts your sleep. People with sleep apnea may cycle through this disruptive pattern dozens or even hundreds of times a night.

In obstructive sleep apnea, the most common form of sleep apnea, the throat muscles relax while you're asleep, closing your airway. Another form known as central sleep apnea occurs when the brain fails to send the proper signal to the muscles that control breathing. You can have either condition or a combination of both. This condition is quite common. According to the American Sleep Apnea Association, twelve million Americans know that they have sleep apnea, and another ten million are undiagnosed.

Signs of sleep apnea include hypersomnia (excessive daytime sleepiness), waking up with a dry mouth or sore throat, morning headaches, insomnia, and loud snoring. Yet people with sleep apnea may not realize that they have it until their sleeping partners point out that they're not breathing during the night.

A Continuous Positive Airway Pressure machine (CPAP) is the most common treatment for sleep apnea. This device includes a mask or nosepiece that is connected to a machine by a hose. This hose supplies a steady stream of pressurized air that keeps your airway open for breathing. While it may take some getting used to, a CPAP machine can have a positive, noticeable effect on your quality of sleep and how rested you feel during the day.

Other treatment options include custom-made mouthguards and surgery. Again, talk to your doctor if you have the symptoms of sleep apnea.

- *Nighttime Heartburn*

Heartburn is a condition with a misleading name. It isn't an affliction of the heart at all but an irritation of the esophagus.

It occurs when stomach acid seeps upward through the lower esophageal sphincter (LES), causing an unpleasant burning sensation. It affects about twenty million people, 80 percent of whom experience symptoms at night, which interferes with sleep.

If heartburn symptoms are keeping you awake, avoid large meals and heavy snacks in the evening and have your last meal several hours before bedtime. Limiting known heartburn triggers like alcohol, tomatoes, citrus fruits, and spicy foods is also smart. Don't smoke because it relaxes the LES and stimulates the production of stomach acid, both of which aggravate heartburn symptoms.

Diet may play a bigger role in heartburn than you realize. A growing body of evidence suggests that the excessive amount of carbohydrates in our diets (starchy foods, chips, sugars, and junk foods) is damaging to our nervous systems. This constant barrage can result in excessive acid production, which leads to heartburn. Reducing carbohydrate intake to fewer than one hundred grams per day can reduce and often reverse excessive acid production.

A natural antacid like deglycyrrhizinated licorice, slippery elm, or aloe vera juice (gel) can help ease stomach discomfort. Elevating your head six to eight inches to keep acid from flowing into your esophagus works well. Sleeping on your left side can also help reduce symptoms.

Finally, heartburn can often be the result of an over dominant, sympathetic nervous system. The vagus nerve represents the main component of the parasympathetic nervous system and is responsible for several functions, including mood, heart rate, immunity, and digestion. If other measures don't work, therapy to help balance the nervous system can often bring relief and ultimately resolve the underlying problem. If your heartburn symptoms persist or worsen, talk to your doctor to rule out something more serious.

- *Narcolepsy*

When the brain fails to regulate the wake-sleep cycles, it can manifest as a neurological disorder known as narcolepsy. Someone with narcolepsy will fall asleep and awaken while he or she is still in REM sleep. That person also experiences involuntary fragments of REM sleep during the day. During this phase of sleep, his or her muscles are in a state of paralysis. This is the reason that narcolepsy is associated with an inability to move. Although narcoleptics are constantly sleepy, they don't sleep any more than the average person. They simply have no control over when and where it occurs.

Signs of narcolepsy include excessive daytime sleepiness (You may fall asleep with no notice while driving or eating, for example) and cataplexy, a sudden loss of muscle tone. Cataplexy can be triggered by emotions such as laughter, anger, or surprise. You suddenly experience limb weakness, like having your knees buckle or dropping something for no reason. You may have hallucinations or bizarre dreams while falling asleep because you're slipping right into REM sleep. You may have sleep paralysis, which is the temporary inability to move your body during sleep-wake transitions. You may have leg spasms and nighttime restlessness.

Researchers aren't sure what causes narcolepsy, but factors like brain injuries, autoimmune disorders, infections, or low levels of histamines (substances in the blood that promote wakefulness) may play a role. Other factors may include environmental toxins such as pesticides, weed killers, heavy metals, and secondhand smoke. If you think that you may have narcolepsy, keep a sleep diary and talk to your doctor about the symptoms you're having.

Treat Sleep as a Necessity and Not as a Luxury

So what's the takeaway here? Sleep is as essential to good health as any other aspect of the *Extinguish the Flame Program*. Just as better nutrition leads to better sleep and vice versa, quality sleep and quality life go hand in hand.

Getting enough sleep will help reduce inflammation throughout your body, help you stay healthy, and give you sustained energy to tackle your day.

Chapter 10
Smart Supplementation

Step Six of the Extinguish the Flame Program

> *Millions of Americans today are taking dietary supplements, practicing yoga, and integrating other natural therapies into their lives. These are all preventive measures that will keep them out of the doctor's office and drive down the costs of treating serious problems like heart disease and diabetes.*
>
> *- Andrew Weil, MD, physician and author*

Now that you understand the importance of sleep and are hopefully on the road to better quality sleep yourself, let's look at the final step of the *Extinguish the Flame Program*: smart supplementation. Here's the thing. Sometimes, it's difficult to get all of the nutrients that your body needs, even with the most impeccable and healthiest of diets. This is why supplementation is important, especially if you're combatting a lot of inflammation.

There are hundreds, if not thousands, of vitamins, minerals, and phytonutrients on which the body thrives, and we're only now beginning to understand some of the complex interplay of all of these nutrients. However, the *Extinguish the Flame Program* focuses on the specific vitamins, minerals, and supplements that have the highest impact on inflammation and overall health.

You'll note that I haven't included specific dosages or recommended amounts of these supplements. You should talk to your nutrition-oriented healthcare provider about the supplements and amounts that are most appropriate for you.

My goal is to educate you about the supplements that will be the most effective and that you may want to include as part of your overall regime.

Vitamins and Minerals

- *Vitamin C*

Vitamin C is one of the best-known antioxidants. It's used for the growth and repair of tissues throughout the body. It aids in maintaining healthy teeth and bones, repairing wounds, and preventing plaque buildup in your arteries, which can lead to heart disease and a stroke. It may help prevent high blood pressure, common colds, osteoarthritis, asthma, and preeclampsia. It may decrease blood sugar in people with diabetes and improve vision.

New research is testing the impact of high doses of intravenous vitamin C. It appears that it may help to slow the spread of some types of cancers and rev up the immune system.

Fruits and vegetables, including citrus fruits, strawberries, kiwi, cantaloupe, tomatoes, potatoes, red and green peppers, broccoli, and Brussels sprouts, are all excellent sources of vitamin C. However, taking a supplement can make sure you're getting enough vitamin C to help fight inflammation. One of my favorites is organic acerola berry, which contains the highest level of naturally occurring vitamin C along with additional nutrients.

- *Vitamin D3*

Did you know that nearly half of all people in the world are deficient in vitamin D? Vitamin D is necessary to build healthy bones and muscles because your body uses it to absorb calcium. It helps prevent osteoporosis (thinning of the bones), and it is necessary for immune function and cognitive brain support. Few foods contain vitamin D, so you need to get it in the form of sun exposure and, or supplements. If you live in the northern part of the country, you may need additional supplementation, especially during the winter months. The good thing is that it is easy to find these supplements in both animal and vegan forms.

It can be tempting to choose the supplements that you think may be the most beneficial, but I strongly urge you to make the decisions with the support and guidance of your healthcare provider. Consider Jessica's story. She was alrea-dy taking some supplements, but they weren't helping her overall health.

Choosing the Right Supplements

Jessica, 58, had been diagnosed with rheumatoid arthritis and severe muscle atrophy. She had been experiencing excruciating pain for the last several years and could not raise her hands above her shoulders. Her rheumatologist told her she had severe joint damage and had her taking large doses of Prednisone, a steroid, and a non-steroidal anti-inflammatory drug, but was urging her to take much stronger drugs. Jessica was already following an anti-inflammatory, gluten-free, dairy-free, and soy-free diet and was taking several supplements.

Despite the anti-inflammatory diet, her blood test for C-reactive protein (CRP) was 50 mg/ml (a normal level of 3 mg/ml), and her female hormones were out of balance. I had her add vitamin D, colostrum, and butyric acid supplements to her daily regime. By her next visit, her pain was 90 percent gone, and she could raise her hands over her head, and she was thrilled that she finally had a handle on this chronic disease. A blood test revealed that her CRP had dropped from 50 to less than 4.5!

Drew Collins, ND

- *Magnesium*

This mineral is a natural muscle relaxant, and it can help ease you into the first stage of sleep. It's used by the body to produce energy, and it helps with healthy nerve and muscle function, including maintaining heart rhythm. Green leafy vegetables (like spinach), legumes, nuts (especially cashews), seeds, and whole grains (gluten-free if you have gluten sensitivity or intolerance) are all good sources of magnesium, yet most people don't get enough magnesium in their diets.

If you take magnesium, try taking it about thirty minutes before bedtime to help you get to sleep. There are many good forms of magnesium, including glycinate, malate, and citrate. One of my favorites is magnesium threonate, which crosses the blood-brain barrier, providing cognitive support and inducing a calming effect.

Other Supplements

- *5-HTP*

5-HTP, which stands for 5-hydroxytryptophan, is a precursor to tryptophan, an amino acid that appears to increase the good-mood brain chemical serotonin. 5-HTP can help people sleep, and therefore, it is used to treat insomnia, as well as depression, anxiety, migraines, and fibromyalgia. It may also be helpful in treating premenstrual syndrome, premenstrual dysphoric disorder, attention deficit hyperactivity disorder, and seizure disorder. New research also suggests that it may help reduce appetite and caloric intake in the obese because of its impact on serotonin.

- *Astaxanthin*

Known as one of the world's most powerful antioxidants, astaxanthin is a carotenoid found in nature, primarily in marine organisms such as microalgae, salmon, trout, krill, shrimp, crayfish, and crustaceans. Astaxanthin is six thousand times more powerful than vitamin C, one hundred times more powerful than vitamin E, and five times more powerful than beta-carotene in its ability to quench free radicals that damage our healthy cells. It has well-documented anti-inflammatory and immune-stimulating effects. Numerous studies support the use of astaxanthin to decrease the risk of certain chronic diseases. Since astaxanthin is able to go directly to the brain by crossing the blood-brain barrier, it may also reduce oxidative stress in the nervous system, which further reduces the risk of neurodegenerative diseases like Alzheimer's and Parkinson's disease.

- *Boswellia*

The Boswellia tree, which is native to the Middle East and North Africa, produces compounds that have been used in anti-inflammatory healing for thousands of years. Boswellia is great on its own, but when coupled with the curcuminoids (the active ingredients) of turmeric, it may be even more effective at supporting the immune system and reducing inflammation. Boswellia has been reported to help treat various conditions, including osteoporosis, rheumatoid arthritis, ulcerative colitis, irritable bowel syndrome, and bronchitis. It also reduces the risk of developing asthma.

- *Coenzyme Q10*

Coenzyme Q10 (CoQ10) is similar to a vitamin that is found in every cell of the body. It also functions as an antioxidant, which protects the body from damage and inflammation. Your body uses it for cell growth and maintenance. CoQ10 improves immune function and may help treat heart disease, high blood pressure, migraines, and diabetes.

Oily fish like salmon and tuna, organ meats like liver, and whole grains all contain CoQ10. You'll also find it in different forms of supplements, including soft-gel capsules, tablets, and oral sprays. If you are on statin drugs for lowering cholesterol, make sure to consider taking CoQ10 because statins deplete the body of CoQ10. It is important to discuss this with your health practitioner.

- *Fish Oil*

There's nothing fishy about fish oil. Fish oil seems to help improve neurotransmitter function in the brain. It may help conditions such as Alzheimer's disease, traumatic brain injury, dementia, and attention deficit disorder.

Fish oil contains omega-3 fats, which are linked to preventing and easing depression, decreasing unhealthy triglycerides, and reducing inflammation in joints. While it's found in fatty fish and nuts, including walnuts, supplementing can make it easier to get more omega-3 fats into your diet.

You'll find fish oil supplements in both soft gel capsules and liquid form. Specific liquid versions have improved absorption, are tasty (I'm a fan of the fruit-flavored version for children and those who object to any amount of fish oil scent or taste), and are a smart choice if you have difficulty swallowing large capsules. Double-check the potency and purity of the supplements you choose, and make sure that they're free of heavy metals like mercury and other contaminants.

> ***Treating a Variety of Symptoms with Supplements***
> Ginny, 67, had been suffering from a number of symptoms — fatigue, hot flashes, joint pain, poor memory and headaches. Testing showed high toxicity and inflammation. She modified the ketogenic diet she had been following and started taking supplements, including fish oil, vitamin D, methylated B vitamins, and magnesium.
>
> Two months later, she felt much better, and all of her symptoms improved. Her follow-up blood test revealed that her toxicity and inflammation markers were normal.
>
> - Diana Fatayerji, PhD

- *Ginger*

Ginger is a flowering plant that is related to turmeric. Its active ingredient, gingerol, has been shown to be a highly effective antioxidant and anti-inflammatory agent. It provides relief for indigestion and nausea, and it is a proven pain reliever after intense exercise. Gingerol is also shown to help improve cardiovascular disease, type-2 diabetes, and overall gastrointestinal function and health.

- *Prebiotics, Probiotics, and Postbiotics*

Probiotics are living organisms that can help improve a variety of health conditions. Prebiotics help feed the beneficial bacteria in your gut, while probiotics are beneficial bacteria. Because they help restore and maintain healthy gut flora, they can be particularly helpful after taking antibiotics or other medications that throw off your gut's natural balance. It's not only antibiotics that can do this. One study found that women who took oral contraceptives for more than five years were three times more likely to develop the inflammatory digestive disorder Crohn's disease than women who did not.

Prebiotics and probiotics work together, and they may prevent relapsing gastroenteritis, inflammatory bowel disease, and irritable bowel syndrome. They may help treat rheumatoid arthritis, liver disease, and diabetes. These organisms can help ease diarrhea. They can also aid in the prevention of atopic eczema, respiratory infections in children, and cavities. Recent research suggests that they may also help lower cholesterol, regulate the immune system, and reduce the risk of depression.

Foods including onions, garlic, bananas, beans, asparagus, Jerusalem artichokes, mushrooms, chicory root, and soluble tapioca fiber are all good sources of prebiotics, which feed the healthy bacteria in the large intestine. Yogurt, aged cheeses, and kefir contain probiotics, but be careful about these sources if you're allergic or sensitive to dairy products. As mentioned in previous chapters, A2/A2 kefir and yogurt dairy products are similar to mothers' milk and, as a result, may be an alternative choice. Other probiotic foods include kimchi, sauerkraut, miso, tempeh, and kombucha. You can also buy prebiotics and probiotics in supplement form.

Postbiotics are a broad term used to describe the metabolic byproducts or substances produced by the action of probiotics (beneficial bacteria) during the fermentation process. These byproducts include various compounds such as short-chain fatty acids, peptides, organic acids, enzymes, and other bioactive substances.

Unlike probiotics and prebiotics, postbiotics refer to the compounds that are generated as a result of the metabolic activity of these microorganisms.

Research suggests that postbiotics may also contribute to the health-promoting effects associated with probiotics. They can influence the immune system, help regulate inflammation, and support the overall balance of the gut microbiota. Additionally, postbiotics are considered nonliving bacteria that are generated during the fermentation or growth of probiotics. Postbiotics are stable and do not require refrigeration, making them potentially more convenient for certain applications.

Common sources of postbiotics include fermented foods like yogurt, kefir, sauerkraut, kimchi, and fermented coconut water, where the fermentation process produces these beneficial compounds. The study of postbiotics is a new but rapidly evolving area in the field of gut health and microbiome research. Postbiotics are also available in supplement form.

- *Butyrate*

Butyrate is a type of short-chain fatty acid (SCFA). It is one of the beneficial postbiotics produced by the gut microbiota during the fermentation of dietary fibers.

Butyrate plays a crucial role in maintaining gut health and overall well-being. It serves as the primary energy source for the cells lining the colon, supporting their proper function and integrity. Additionally, butyrate is known for its anti-inflammatory properties and is associated with the regulation of immune responses in the gastrointestinal tract.

Consuming a diet rich in fiber, especially from sources like whole grains (remember to avoid gluten-containing grains if you have a sensitivity, intolerance, or celiac disease) and certain vegetables, can contribute to the production of butyrate by the gut microbiota. The presence of adequate butyrate is often considered beneficial for promoting a healthy gut environment and supporting various aspects of digestive and immune health. Butyrate (Butyric acid) is available in supplement form.

- *Resveratrol*

You've probably heard that resveratrol, the antioxidant found in red wine, can be good for you. This antioxidant appears to have anti-inflammatory properties. It may help reduce blood sugar levels in people with diabetes, improve immune function, treat acne, and ease allergy symptoms.

Resveratrol may also work to prevent or possibly slow the progression of diseases like Alzheimer's. In a randomized, phase two, placebo-controlled, and double-blind study, resveratrol in concentrated high doses was shown to decrease a biomarker for people with mild to moderate symptoms of Alzheimer's. Resveratrol reduced some of the plaques that produced swelling in the brain but also decreased brain size. While this sounds contradictory in terms of health, understand that Alzheimer's causes inflammation of the brain. If you reduce the inflammation and swelling, the overall size of the brain will possibly diminish.

- *Turmeric*

Turmeric is an antioxidant superfood that is getting a lot more attention from mainstream media today. You can consume it in its natural root form or use powdered turmeric as a spice. You can take it as a capsulized supplement or in a liquid tincture.

Turmeric's active ingredients are called curcuminoids. One of these, called curcumin, has long been studied for its health benefits. It is arguably one of nature's best anti-inflammatory agents. Curcumin has been shown to help reduce inflammation, which may help ease arthritis, anxiety, high cholesterol, metabolic syndrome, and other conditions.

Turmeric has been consumed by Indians for centuries, and it is a staple in Indian cuisine. Although it is not absorbed well by the body, it has an accumulative effect. In other words, taking a little every day will provide benefits. However, because it was introduced to the United States only recently and primarily in the form of supplements, most of us don't have the same accumulative benefit of having grown up consuming it the way Indians have.

If you're going to take a turmeric supplement, look for one that's certified organic (it has been grown without pesticides) and improves bioavailability for better absorption. Because turmeric is a fat-soluble ingredient, it is better taken with healthy fats such as nuts, avocados, or other healthy fats to improve bioavailability.

- *Green Tea and Matcha*

Green tea is a type of tea that is made from Camellia sinensis leaves and buds. The key difference between green tea and other types of tea, such as black or oolong, lies in the minimal oxidation process that green tea undergoes during its production. This process helps preserve the natural compounds and antioxidants found in the tea leaves.

Green tea is loaded with polyphenols, particularly catechins, which act as powerful antioxidants. These compounds help neutralize free radicals in the body, reducing oxidative stress and contributing to overall health. Regular consumption of green tea has been associated with a lower risk of cardiovascular diseases. The antioxidants in green tea may help lower levels of bad cholesterol (LDL cholesterol) and improve artery function. The caffeine and amino acid L-theanine present in green tea can have synergistic effects, promoting improved cognitive function, alertness, and mood.

Green tea is available in various forms, providing flexibility in consumption. These include:

- Loose Leaf Tea can be steeped in hot water to make a refreshing and aromatic beverage.

- Pre-packaged tea bags offer convenience and ease of use. Simply steep the tea bag in hot water for a few minutes.

Green tea extracts are concentrated forms of the active compounds in green tea. They are available in supplement form and can be consumed in controlled doses.

Matcha and regular green tea both come from the Camellia sinensis plant, but the way they are grown and harvested differs significantly, leading to distinct differences in flavor, texture, and nutritional content.

About 20-30 days before harvest, matcha tea plants are covered with shade cloths to block around 90% of sunlight. This increases chlorophyll production, boosts amino acids, and gives the leaves a darker green color.

Only the youngest and most tender leaves are picked by hand, ensuring high quality. After harvesting, the leaves are steamed to prevent oxidation, which helps retain their vibrant green color and nutritional content. The leaves are then dried and sorted. The dried leaves, known as tencha, are ground into a fine powder using traditional stone mills.

- *Mushrooms*

The term "Shroom Boom" is associated with the increasing recognition of the health benefits offered by certain mushrooms, particularly those known for their anti-inflammatory properties.

Mushrooms have a rich history in traditional medicine, and recent research has illuminated their potential contributions to overall health. These fungi contain bioactive compounds such as polysaccharides and polyphenols, which demonstrate anti-inflammatory effects by modulating the immune system and regulating inflammatory responses. Noteworthy mushrooms in this regard include reishi, known as the "king of mushrooms" (reishi has been recognized as a medicinal mushroom for over 2000 years, having a long history of promoting health, immune support, and longevity in Asia), shiitake, maitake with potential immune-boosting properties, and cordyceps recognized for its adaptogenic, and energizing qualities. Turkey tail and chaga are also valued for their immunomodulatory and antioxidant-rich profiles. Other healthy mushrooms include lion's mane, known for its cognitive boosting properties, tremella for its ability to support collagen production for healthy skin, and antrodia for its liver protection properties. When looking for mushroom extracts, be certain to look for those with the highest level of the most common active ingredients in the mushroom, known as beta 1:3-1:6 glucans. While there are a variety of additional mushrooms with health benefits, I have listed some of the most common.

Incorporating a variety of these mushrooms into one's diet can be a flavorful and nutritious way to support overall health and align with the growing interest in the "Shroom Boom" trend. Whether enjoyed in meals or as supplements, mushrooms provide a natural source of beneficial compounds that contribute to holistic well-being. It's advisable to consult with a healthcare provider for personalized advice on incorporating mushrooms, especially for individuals with specific health concerns or conditions.

- *Glutathione*

Glutathione is a powerful antioxidant naturally produced in the body. It plays a crucial role in various physiological processes, including detoxification, immune function, and cellular defense against oxidative stress. Research has indicated several potential benefits of glutathione supplementation: Glutathione helps protect the liver from damage caused by heavy metals, pollutants, alcohol, and drugs. It binds to toxins, allowing the body to eliminate them. It is essential for a healthy immune system and helps the body fight off infections and diseases. Glutathione helps to reduce oxidative damage and inflammation in the brain and may play a role in protecting against neurological disorders such as Parkinson's and Alzheimer's disease. Glutathione is available in intravenous therapy (IV) and oral supplementation, and it is known as reduced glutathione.

While there is promising evidence supporting the benefits of glutathione supplementation, it's important to note that more research is needed to fully understand its effects on human health. Additionally, the effectiveness of glutathione supplements can vary depending on factors such as dosage, formulation, and individual health status. It's always advisable to consult with a healthcare provider before starting any new supplement regimen.

- *Olive Oil*

Olive oil is known for its anti-inflammatory properties and has been associated with various health benefits, including the reduction of inflammation. The key components responsible for these anti-inflammatory effects are the presence of monounsaturated fats, particularly oleic acid, and hydroxytyrosol in olive oil.

Oleic acid has been shown to have anti-inflammatory and antioxidant properties. Additionally, extra virgin olive oil (EVOO), which is less processed and retains more of the natural compounds from olives, contains polyphenols with anti-inflammatory effects. Hydroxytyrosol, one of the main active ingredients in olive oil, has been shown in studies to reduce the risk of cardiovascular disease.

A study published in the "Journal of Agricultural and Food Chemistry" in 2017 examined the impact of hydroxytyrosol on blood lipids and markers of oxidative stress in individuals at high risk of cardiovascular disease. The results suggested that supplementation with hydroxytyrosol may help improve lipid profiles and reduce oxidative stress, both of which are important factors in cardiovascular health.

Furthermore, a systematic review and meta-analysis published in "Critical Reviews in Food Science and Nutrition" in 2020 evaluated the cumulative evidence from various studies on the cardiovascular effects of hydroxytyrosol. The analysis concluded that hydroxytyrosol consumption was associated with significant reductions in markers of inflammation and oxidative stress, as well as improvements in endothelial (inside lining of blood vessels) function and blood lipid profiles, all of which contribute to a lower risk of cardiovascular disease.

While these findings are promising, more research is needed to fully understand the mechanisms underlying the cardiovascular benefits of hydroxytyrosol and to determine optimal doses for therapeutic use. Additionally, it's essential to consider other factors in the Mediterranean diet, of which olive oil is a key component, that may contribute synergistically to its cardio-protective effects.

The anti-inflammatory benefits of olive oil are often linked to its potential impact on several inflammatory markers and pathways within the body. Incorporating olive oil into a balanced and healthy diet may contribute to managing inflammation and reducing the risk of chronic inflammatory conditions. Recent studies have shown that these powerful ingredients may decrease the risk of Metabolic syndrome, a group of conditions that together raise your risk of coronary heart disease and diabetes.

- *Colostrum*

Colostrum, often referred to as "first milk," is produced by mammals, including humans, in the initial days following birth. It's packed with essential nutrients, antibodies, and growth factors, providing numerous benefits, especially for newborns. Some of the proven benefits of colostrum include:

- Nutrient-rich: Colostrum is rich in proteins, carbohydrates, fats, vitamins, and minerals, providing essential nutrients necessary for the growth and development of newborns.
- Antibodies and immune factors: Colostrum contains high levels of antibodies such as Immunoglobulin A (IgA), Immunoglobulin G (IgG), and Immunoglobulin M (IgM), which help boost the newborn's

immune system and protect against infections and diseases.
- Growth factors: Colostrum contains growth factors such as insulin-like growth factor 1 (IGF-1) and transforming growth factors (TGFs), which promote tissue repair, growth, and development.
- Digestive benefits: Colostrum contains bioactive compounds like lactoferrin and lactoperoxidase, which support digestive health by promoting the growth of beneficial bacteria in the gut and protectting against harmful pathogens.
- Anti-inflammatory properties: Components in colostrum, such as cytokines and interleukins, possess anti-inflammatory properties, which can help reduce inflammation and support overall immune function.
- Enhanced nutrient absorption: Colostrum contains factors that aid in the absorption of nutrients, making it easier for newborns to digest and utilize nutrients from breast milk or formula.
- Gut health: Colostrum supports the development of a healthy gut microbiome, which is essential for proper digestion, nutrient absorption, and immune function.
- Protective effects: Studies suggest that colostrum may have protective effects against conditions such as diarrhea, respiratory infections, allergies, and inflammatory bowel diseases.
- Promotes brain development: Components found in colostrum, such as growth factors and fatty acids, are essential for brain development and may contribute to cognitive function in newborns.
- Wound healing: Colostrum contains factors that promote tissue repair and wound healing, making it beneficial for newborns, especially those born prematurely or with low birth weight.

Overall, colostrum plays a crucial role in providing essential nutrients, antibodies, and growth factors that support the health, growth, and development of newborns.

Before You Supplement Your Diet

As you can see, a number of supplements have been proven to help fight inflammation in your body. Talk with your nutrition-oriented healthcare provider about the ones that may be right for you and the appropriate dosages. He or she will keep your current health and goals in mind when determining the ones that will be of the most benefit to you.

Chapter 11
Extinguish the Flame for Life

Keeping Inflammation at Bay

You can take steps today to help stack the odds in your favor to optimize your genetic potential.

- Bruce Howe DC, CCN, author

You've now learned not only how damaging inflammation is to your body but how to fight it by making lifestyle changes to help extinguish its flame. As you read the previous chapters, you may have realized that you're already taking some steps to help fight inflammation. Maybe you already make sleep a priority or exercise regularly. Maybe you embrace gratitude as part of your daily life.

My goal in writing this book wasn't to force you to make a sweeping lifestyle change that you can't maintain. I wanted to educate you about what you can do to help protect your health, no matter what challenges you may face.

As I said in the introduction, I've been studying inflammation, its impact on overall health, and ways that we can fight it for decades. Now, as I am in my seventies, I realize that it truly has become my life's work. I'm honored and grateful when I learn of the impact these kinds of dietary and lifestyle modifications have had on people. Earlier in this book, you heard from some of the doctors who have used similar anti-inflammatory strategies with their patients, but I also want you to hear from people who have benefited by taking baby steps toward improving their overall health.

> "I'm fifty-seven, and I have been on high blood pressure medication for seventeen years. Five months ago, I tried a supplement containing turmeric, Boswellia, and ginger extracts for inflammation in my knee," says John. "I discovered that this product not only helps with inflammation but also has reduced my blood pressure. I now take three capsules a day and no longer take any prescription drugs for high blood pressure. I was also diagnosed with gout and have been fighting that for the last seventeen years. So, I have not had a gout attack either."
>
> Cindy told us about the success she'd had with specific nutritional products. "I started a nutrition program in April 2017 under the guidance of my doctor in Dunwoody, Georgia," she says.
>
> "Since starting, my biggest accomplishment has been getting off all my medications for diabetes and blood pressure and actually reversing my diabetes...I started walking and could only do about fifteen minutes a day. Now, I walk an average of five miles a day and have participated in several 5Ks...I've lost 129 pounds since I started, and I'm doing things now I would have never done before because I was so self-conscious. For example, I went paddle boarding this summer, and the old me would have never done this!"

Attitude Gratitude, Find a Way to Be a Blessing to Others Everyday
Bruce Howe, DC CCN author

I have come to understand that this is my journey and that God has bigger plans for me. I appreciate each and every breath that I take and every moment I am alive. I am constantly reminded that we get to live in the moment and that we do not know what the future holds.

Each morning and evening, I take a gratitude walk. During this time, I get outside (rain or shine) and thank God for the simple things I take for granted: the ability to put my feet on the ground, witness His beautiful creation, to hear the birds chirp and children laugh, to smell the ocean air, to experience the touch of a warm embrace, and to taste the sweetness of a crisp, juicy apple. It is a time when I ask God to help me be a blessing to others every day.

Without the devastating effects of cancer and the treatment I underwent, I would not have been able to share my story or impact someone else's life along the way. That's why I wrote this book. It's my hope that it will have a positive impact on your journey in life as well.

You can't control every aspect of your life. As you just learned, cancer can strike even the healthiest of people. But you can take steps today and from here on out that will help stack the odds in your favor. You can do your best to optimize your genetic potential. You may not adopt every aspect of the *Extinguish the Flame Program*, but every small change you make can make a difference in not only how you feel today but also how long and well you live. After all, you have but one body and one life. Don't you want to do everything you can to live, love, and embrace every aspect of it? Here's to your good health!

Get in Touch

I would like to give my sincere thanks to you for your interest in this book. Have you found it helpful? Have you noticed an improvement in your health since you started following the *Extinguish the Flame Program*? Do you want to share your own experience with me? Please feel free to get in touch with me at drhowe@hotmail.com.

- Bruce Howe, DC, CCN

Notes

Chapter 1
Centers for Disease Control and Prevention, "Sleep and Sleep Disorders,"

https://www.cdc.gov/sleep/index.html.

Lack of Exercise Is a Major Cause of Chronic Diseases. FW Booth, Ph.D., CK Roberts, Ph.D., MJ Lave, Ph.D. Comprehensive Physiology. 2(2): 1143-1211. April 2012.

Mental Health in Adolescents. U.S. Department of Health & Human Services Office of Adolescent Health.

https://www.hhs.gov/ash/oah/adolescent-development/mental-health/index.html Accessed July 31, 2018.

Help for Mental Illnesses. NIH National Institute of Mental Health. https://www.nimh.nih.gov/health/find-help/index.shtml Accessed July 31, 2018.

"Journal of Neuroinflammation" July 28, 2022, Article number 193 (2022).

UC Berkeley School of Public Health March 1, 2023 by Sheila Kaplan

Mendoza-Martínez, V. M., Zavala-Solares, M. R., Espinosa-Flores, A. J., León-Barrera, K. L., Alcántara-Suárez, R., Carrillo-Ruíz, J. D., Escobedo, G., Roldan-Valadez, E., Esquivel-Velázquez, M., Meléndez-Mier, G., & Bueno-Hernández, N. (2022). Is a Non-Caloric Sweetener-Free Diet Good to Treat Functional Gastro-intestinal Disorder

Symptoms? A Randomized Cont-rolled Trial. Nutrients, 14(5), 1095.

https://doi.org/10.3390/nu14051095

Chandra V, Pandav R, Dodge HH, Johnston JM, Belle SH, De-Kosky ST, et al. Incidence of Alzheimer's disease in rural community in India: the Indo-US study. Neurology. 2001; 57 (6):985-9.

Chapter 2

What is Healthy Weight Loss? Centers for Disease Control and Prevention.

https://www.cdc.gov/healthyweight/losing_weight/index.html February 13, 2018.

Where people around the world eat the most sugar and fat. RA Ferdman. The Washington Post. February 5, 2015.

Weight management. NIH National Institute of Diabetes and Digestive and Kidney Diseases.

https://www.niddk.nih.gov/health-information/weight-management. Accessed July 31, 2018.

Low-grade inflammation, diet composition and health: current research evidence and its translation. AM Minihane et al. British Journal of Nutrition. 114(7); 999-1012. October 14, 2015.

The Anti-Inflammatory Diet: A Way to Manage Chronic Pain. Online health chat with William Welchese, DO, PhD, and Carla Vanpelt, PCC.

https://my.clevelandclinic.org/health/transcripts/2748_the-anti-inflammatory-diet-a-way-to-manage-chronic-pain July 13, 2015.

Dr. Weil's Anti-Inflammatory Food Pyramid. Dr. Andrew Weil.

https://www.drweil.com/diet-nutrition/anti-inflammatory-diet-pyramid/dr-weils-anti-inflammatory-food-pyramid/ Accessed August 6, 2018.

Survey: Stress in America Increases for the First Time in 10 Years. David Oliver. U.S. News and World Report.

https://health.usnews.com/wellness/health-buzz/articles/2017-02-15/survey-stress-in-america-increases-for-the-first-time-in-10-years Accessed August 6, 2018.

Eight in 10 Americans Afflicted by Stress. Gallup Poll. https://news.gallup.com/poll/224336/eight-americans-afflicted-stress.aspx December 20, 2017.

Waist-to-height ratio index for predicting incidences of hypertension: the ARIRANG study. JR Choi, SB Koh, and E Choi. BMC Public Health. 18:767. 2018.

Waist-to-height ratio, inflammation and CVD risk in obese children. J Olza et al. Public Health & Nutrition. 17(10):2378-85. October 2014.

Body mass index, waist circumference, and waist-to-height ratio for prediction of multiple metabolic risk factors in Chinese elderly population. G Zhan et al. Science Reports. 8: 385. January 10, 2018.

Inflammatory Bowel Diseases, Volume 24, Issue 5: 1005-1020. April 23, 2018.

Sleep Disorders and Sleep Deprivation: An Unmet Public Health Problem. Institute of Medicine. Washington, DC: The National Academies Press; 2006.

Inc, G. (2022, June 28). World Unhappier, More Stressed Out Than Ever. Gallup.com.

https://news.gallup.com/poll/394025/world-unhappier-stressed-ever.aspxh

What doctors wish patients knew about insomnia. (2022, May 13). American Medical Association.

https://www.ama-assn.org/delivering-care/public-health/what-doctors-wish-patients-knew-about-insomnia

Centers for Disease Control and Prevention. (2022, August 26). Adults - Sleep and Sleep Disorders | CDC. Www.cdc.gov.

https://www.cdc.gov/sleep/data-and-statistics/adults.html

Find out how many hours of sleep you need to feel your best. (2020, December 21). Healthline.

https://www.healthline.com/nutrition/how-much-sleep-you-need

https://water.usgs.gov/nawqa/pnsp/usage/maps/show_map.php?year=2018&map=PARAQUAT&hilo=L

https://www.epa.gov/sites/default/files/2019-03/documents/paraquat-dichloride-one-sip-can-kill-3-8-19.pdf

https://www.publiceye.ch/fileadmin/doc/Pestizide/Paraquat_Leaks/1983_ScienceDigest_ParaquatWeedKillerisKillingPeople.pdf

https://www.nih.gov/news-events/news-releases/nih-study-finds-two-pesticides-associated-parkinsons-disease

https://www.epa.gov/pesticide-worker-safety/paraquat-dichloride-training-certified-applicators

https://time.com/4089310/sugar-effects/

Chapter 4

Inflammation and its discontents: the role of cytokines in the pathophysiology of major depression. Miller et al. Biological Psychiatry. 65(9): 732-41. May 1, 2009.

Cytokines and cognition: the case for a head-to-toe inflammatory paradigm. Wilson et al. JAGS. 50:2041-2056. 2002.

A randomized controlled trial of the tumor necrosis factor antagonist infliximab for treatment-resistant depression: the role of baseline inflammatory biomarkers. CL Raison et al. JAMA Psychiatry. 70:31-41. January 2013.

Chapter 5

EWG's 2018 Shopper's Guide to Pesticides in Produce. S Lunder. EWG. April 20, 2018.

https://www.ewg.org/foodnews/summary.php

Cleaning Supplies and Household Chemicals. American Lung Association. Accessed August 7, 2018.

http://www.lung.org/our-initiatives/healthy-air/indoor/indoor-air-pollutants/cleaning-supplies-household-chem.html

10 Chemicals to Avoid in your Everyday Products. One Green Planet.

https://www.onegreenplanet.org/lifestyle/chemicals-to-avoid-in-your-everyday-products/ April 3, 2017.

EWG's Skin Deep Cosmetic Database/Shopping Tips. EWG. https://www.ewg.org/skindeep/top-tips-for-safer-products/#.W0eGpi3Mw6gAccessed August 7, 2018.

American Lung Association. (2021, October 6). Tips to Keep Your Lungs Healthy.

Www.lung.org.

https://www.lung.org/lung-health-diseases/wellness/protecting-your-lungs

https://www.epa.gov/environmental-topics

https://www.epa.gov/saferchoice/products

Chapter 6

AHA/ACC guideline on lifestyle management to reduce cardiovascular risk: a report of the American College of Cardiology/American Heart Association Task Force on practice guidelines.

Eckel RH, Jakicic JM, Ard JD, et al. Journal of the American College of Cardiology. 63(25 Pt B):2960-2984. 2014.

Nutrition and cardiovascular and metabolic diseases. Mozaffarian D. in: Mann DL, Zipes DP, Libby P, Bonow RO, Braunwald E, eds. Braunwald's Heart Disease: A Textbook of Cardiovascular Medicine. 10th ed. Philadelphia, PA: Elsevier Saunders; chap 46. 2015.

Hidden sugars. IHS. Division of Diabetes Treatment and Prevention.
https://www.ihs.gov/MedicalPrograms/Diabetes/HomeDocs/Resources/InstantDownloads/HiddenSugars_508c.pdf January, 2012.

What are added sugars? United States Department of Agriculture. https://www.choosemyplate.gov/what-are-added-sugarsNovember 9, 2016.

Sweet Stuff: How Sugars and Sweeteners Affect Your Health. National Institutes of Health.

https://newsinhealth.nih.gov/2014/10/sweet-stuff October, 2014.

U.S. Drinking Water Widely Contaminated, Taryn Luntz, Scientific American.com December 14, 2009

The Circadian Code, Satchin Panda PhD, June 12, 2018

Chapter 7

Effect of exercise training on chronic inflammation. KM Beavers, TE Brinkley, and BJ Nicklas. Clinica Chimica Acta. 411(0); 785-793. February 25, 2010.

Mild Dehydration Affects Mood in Healthy Young Women. LE Armstrong et al. The Journal of Nutrition. 142(2):382-8. Feb 2012.

Patterns of Sedentary Behavior and Mortality in U.S. Middle-Aged and Older Adults: A National Cohort Study. Annals of Internal Medicine. K. Diaz et al. 167(7): 465-475. September 12, 2017.

Using Pedometers to Increase Physical Activity and Improve Health: A Systematic Review. DM Bravata, MD, et al. JAMA. 298(19): 2296-2304. November 21, 2007.

U.S. Cohort Differences in Body Composition Outcomes of a 6-Month Pedometer-Based Physical Activity Intervention: The ASUKI Step Study. JR Walker et al. Asian Journal of Sports Medicine. 5(4): e25748. December 2014.

The association between daily steps and health, and the mediating role of body composition: a pedometer-based, cross-sectional study in an employed South African population. JD Pillay et al. BMC Public Health. 15:174. February 22, 2015.

Ability to sit and rise from the floor as a predictor of all-cause mortality. L Barbosa, B de Brito et al. European Journal of Preventive Cardiology. 21(7): 892-898. July 1, 2014.

Chapter 8

A comparison of the cardiovascular effects of simulated and spontaneous laughter. MM Law, EA Broadbent, JJ Sollers.

Complementary Therapies in Medicine. 37:103-109. April 2018.

Therapeutic Benefits of Laughter in Mental Health: A Theoretical Review. J Yim. Tohuku Journal of Experimental Medicine. 239(3): 243-9. July 2016.

The power of love: how relationships benefit body and mind." J McIntosh. Medical News Today.

https://www.medicalnewstoday.com/articles/289386.php February 12, 2015.

Inflammation: depression fans the flames and feasts on the heat. JK Kiecolt-Glaser, HM Derry, CP Fagundes. American Journal of Psychiatry. 172(11):1075-91. Nov 1, 2015.

Marriage and long-term survival after coronary artery bypass grafting. K King et al. Health Psychology. 31(1): 55-62. January 2012.

Effect of Therapeutic Touch in Patients with Cancer: a Literature Review. A Tabatabaee et al. Medical Archives. 70(2): 142-147. April 2016.

Social Relationships and Depression: Ten-Year Follow-Up from a Nationally Representative Study. AR Teo, H Choi, M Valenstein. *PLOS ONE.* 8(4): e62396. April 30, 2013.

State and trait affectionate communication buffer adults' stress reactions. K Floyd, PM Pauley, and C Hesse. Communication Monographs, 77: 618-636. 2010.

Affectionate communication received from spouses predicts stress hormone levels in healthy adults. K Floyd, S Riforgiate. Communication Monographs. *75:* 351-368. 2008.

Relational affection predicts resting heart rate and free cortisol secretion during acute stress. K Floyd et al. Behavioral Medicine. *32:* 151-156. 2007.

Wouldn't you like 30 mandated days off? Here are the countries with the most vacation days. John Harrington USAToday.com
https://www.usatoday.com/story/money/2019/07/23/paid-time-off-countries-with-the-most-vacation-days-brazil-france/39702323/ Jul.23, 2019

Counting Blessings versus Burdens: An Experimental Investigation of Gratitude and Subjective Well-Being in Daily Life, Robert Emmons, Michael E. McCullough, Journal of Personality and Social Psychology, 2003 Vol 84, No 2, 377-389

Chapter 9

Sleep Loss and Inflammation. J. Mullington, Ph.D. et al. Best Practices and Research in Clinical Endocrinology Metabolism. 24(5): 775-784. October 2010.

Sleep Loss as a Factor to Induce Cellular and Molecular Inflammatory Variations. G Hurtado-Alvarado, et al. Clinical and Developmental Immunology. 2013: 801341. December 3, 2013.

Sleep Deprivation and Deficiency. National Heart, Lung and Blood Institute. https://www.nhlbi.nih.gov/health-topics/sleep-deprivation-and-deficiency Accessed August 11, 2018.

Sleepfoundation.org, Max Hirshkowitz, PhD, February 2, 2015

American Sleep Apnea Association

https://www.sleepapnea.org/

Chapter 10

High-Dose Vitamin C (PDQ) — Health Professional Version. National Cancer Institute.

https://www.cancer.gov/about-cancer/treatment/cam/hp/vitamin-c-pdq December 13, 2017.

Vitamin C. University of Maryland Medical Center. https://www.umms.org/ummc/patients-visitors/health-library/medical-encyclopedia/articles/vitamin-cJanuary 7, 2017.

Clinical Indications for Probiotics: An Overview. B R Goldin and S L Gorbach. 46(2): S96-S100. February 1, 2008.

A Randomized, Double-Blind, Placebo-Controlled Trial of Resveratrol for Alzheimer Disease. RS Turner, MD, PhD et al. Neurology. 85(16): 1383–1391. October 20, 2015.

Resveratrol Impacts Alzheimer's Disease Biomarker. Georgetown University Medical Center.

https://gumc.georgetown.edu/news/Resveratrol-Impacts-Alzheimers-Disease-Biomarker September 11, 2015.

Vitamin D and Health. Harvard T. Chan School of Public Health.

https://www.hsph.harvard.edu/nutritionsource/what-should-you-eat/vitamins/vitamin-d/ Accessed August 11, 2018.

Vitamin D. National Institutes of Health Office of Dietary Supplements.

https://ods.od.nih.gov/factsheets/VitaminD-Consumer/ April 15, 2016.

Magnesium Fact Sheet for Health Professionals. Natio-nal Institutes of Health Office of Dietary Supplements.

https://ods.od.nih.gov/factsheets/Magnesium-HealthProfessional/March 2, 2018.

Clinical Indications for Probiotics: an overview." BR Goldin and SL Gorbach. Clinical Infections Diseases, Vol. 46: Suppl 2: S96-100. Feb 1, 2008.

Probiotics: In Depth. National Center for Complem-entary and Integrative Health.

https://nccih.nih.gov/health/probiotics/introduction.htm October, 2016.

5-HTP. U.S. National Library of Medicine.

https://medlineplus.gov/druginfo/natural/794.html November 30, 2017.

Coenzyme Q-10. National Center for Complementary and Integrative Health.

https://nccih.nih.gov/health/coq10 July 18, 2018.

Coenzyme Q10: The essential nutrient. Journal of Pharmacology and BioAllied Sciences. 3(3): 466-487. Jul-Sep 2011.

Vitamin D Fact Sheet for Professionals. National Institutes of Health Office of Dietary Supplements. https://ods.od.nih.gov/factsheets/VitaminD-HealthProfessional/ March 2, 2018.

Boswellia Serrata, A Potential Antiinflammatory Agent: An Overview. MZ Siddiqui Indian Journal of Pharmaceutical Sciences. 73(3): 255-261. May-Jun 2011.

Frankincense — therapeutic properties. A.R. Mustafa Al-Yasiry and B Kiczorowska. Postepy Hig Med Dosw (online). 70: 380-391. 2016.

Anti-Oxidative and Anti-Inflammatory Effects of Ginger in Health and Physical Activity: Review of Current Evidence. NS Mashhadi, R Ghiasavand, G Askari, M Hariri, L Darvishi, MR Mofid. Indian Journal of Preventive Medicine. 4(Suppl 1): S36–S42. April 2013.

Curcumin: A Review of Its Effects on Human Health. SJ Hewlings and DS Kalman. Foods. 6(10): 92. Oct 2017.

Vitamin C Fact Sheet for Health Professionals. National Institutes of Health Office of Dietary Supplements. https://ods.od.nih.gov/factsheets/VitaminC-HealthProfessional/March 2, 2018.

Resveratrol. U.S. National Library of Medicine.

https://medlineplus.gov/druginfo/natural/307.html December 14, 2017.

Effect of Probiotics on Depression: A Systematic Review and Meta-Analysis of Randomized Controlled Trials. R Huang, K Wang, and J Hu. Nutrients. 8(8): 483. Aug 2016.

Probiotics and Prebiotics: Present Status and Future Perspectives on Metabolic Disorders. JY Yoo and SS Kim. Nutrients. 8(3): 173. March 2016.

Oral contraceptives, reproductive factors, and risk of inflammatory bowel disease. H Khalili, LM Higuchi, AN Ananthakrishnan, et al. Gut. 10: 1136. May 22, 2012.

Neuroprotective mechanisms of astaxanthin: a potential therapeutic role in preserving cognitive function in age and neurodegeneration. S Grimmig, S-H Kim, et al. GeroScience. 39(1): 19-32. Feb 2017.

Quenching Activities of Common Hydrophilic and Lipophilic Antioxidants against Singlet Oxygen Using Chemiluminescence Detection System. Y Nishida et al. Carotenoid Science 11:16-20. 2007.

Ann N Y Acad Sci. Author manuscript; available in PMC 2018 Sep 1. *Published in final edited form as:* Ann N Y Acad Sci. 2017 Sep; 1403(1): 142–149.Published online 2017 Aug 16. doi: 10.1111/nyas.13431PMCID: PMC5664214 NIHMSID: NIHMS885948 PMID: 28815614Resveratrol for Alzheimer's disease Christine Sawda,[1] Charbel Moussa,[1,2] and R. Scott Turner[1,2]Volume 201 | Article ID 2473495 |

https://doi.org/10.1155/2017/2473495

Antioxidant Effects of a Hydroxytyrosol-Based Pharmaceutical Formulation on Body Composition, Metabolic State, and Gene Expression: A Randomized Double-Blinded, Placebo-Controlled Crossover Trial

Carmela Colica,[1] Laura Di Renzo,[2] Domenico Trombetta,[3] Antonella Smeriglio,[3] Sergio Bernardini,[4]Giorgia Cioccoloni,[5] Renata Costa de Miranda,[5,6] Paola Gualtieri,[5] Paola Sinibaldi Salimei,[2] and Antonino De Lorenzo[2]

Chapter 11

Stem cell divisions, somatic mutations, cancer etiology, and cancer prevention, Christian Tomasetti, Lu Li, Bert Vogelstein, Science, March 24, 2017, Vol 355 Issue 6331 pp. 1330-1334

Made in the USA
Las Vegas, NV
08 May 2025